POSTOPERATIVE PAIN

POSTOPERATIVE PAIN

Understanding its nature and how to treat it

Jane Hosking SRN, ONC

Analgesia Sister, Departments of Surgery and Anaesthetics,
University of Sheffield

and

Edward Welchew MB, ChB, FFARCS

Lecturer in Anaesthetics, Department of Anaesthetics,
University of Sheffield

ff

faber and faber

LONDON · BOSTON

First published in 1985
by Faber and Faber Limited
3 Queen Square London WC1N 3AU

Filmset by Goodfellow & Egan Typesetting Ltd
Printed in Great Britain by Butler & Tannner Ltd
Frome, Somerset
All rights reserved

British Library Cataloguing in Publication Data

Hosking, Jane.
Postoperative pain : understanding its nature
and how to treat it.
1. Pain, Postoperative
I. Title   II. Welchew, Edward
617'.01   RD98.4
ISBN 0-571-13538-2

Library of Congress Cataloging in Publication Data

Hosking, Jane.
Postoperative pain.
Includes bibliographies and index.
1. Pain, Postoperative—Chemotherapy. 2. Analgesics.
3. Surgical nursing. I. Welchew, Edward. II. Title.
[DNLM: 1. Analgesics—therapeutic use—handbooks.
2. Analgesics—therapeutic use—nurses' instruction.
3. Pain, Postoperative—drug therapy—handbooks.
4. Pain, Postoperative—drug therapy—nurses' instruction.
WO 39 H826p]
RD98.4 H67   1985   615'.783   85–4454
ISBN 0-571-13538-2 (pbk.)

To Kath for her patience
To Gwilym for his goading

CONTENTS

ACKNOWLEDGEMENTS

We are grateful to our colleagues who helped in so many ways to enable us to put together this book which we hope will help others to provide more effective pain relief for patients.

We thank Jane Osborne for providing the photography as well as the initial sketches from which Mrs Audrey Besterman drew the final artwork and whom we also thank most warmly.

To avoid disturbing patients at their most vulnerable we invited Peter Herbert, Carmel Donnelly, Enrolled Nurse J. Richards and Karen Giddings MCSP to act as models. We are most grateful to them.

Repeated typing of numerous drafts is always a chore! Chris King showed great patience and willingness and we are grateful.

Finally, we thank Miss P.A. Downie FCSP, Medical Editor at Faber and Faber, for originally persuading us to share our experience by writing this book, and who has guided us through the intricacies of turning thoughts into words!

PREFACE

Pain is the commonest reason for referral to a surgeon, and he is expected to provide a cure for it. However, the first and most obvious effect of surgery will be that the patient will probably have even worse pain than before. Effective relief from postoperative pain depends largely on the insight and attitude of those caring directly for the patient.

Understanding the many factors which influence pain, as well as the reasoning behind the prescribing of analgesics, will enable nurses, physiotherapists and others directly involved to develop their essential skills to the advantage of the patient.

Pain is an unpleasant sensation which is usually associated with, and described in terms of, body damage. It is no wonder that patients in pain quickly develop avoidance behaviour and other psychological effects which may adversely affect their postoperative progress, including mobilisation and ability to participate in physiotherapy. Subtle immunological and metabolic changes may make these effects worse, resulting in an increased incidence of chest and urinary infections, worse muscle wasting and poor wound healing.

Each chapter of the book is relatively self-contained, allowing the reader the option of either selecting chapters of particular interest to read first or reading them in order.

Understanding acute pain is vital for the effective management of postoperative patients. This book aims to present a straightforward account of both prescribing information and nursing management, with background information on relevant anatomy, physiology and psychology. It should be of value to all those interested in the care of surgical patients.

Chapter One

THINKING ABOUT PAIN

The interpretation placed on the sensation of pain involves an understanding of both the psychological and the social aspects of pain perception. To some extent all pain is 'in the mind'; rarely is it 'all in the mind'. In the postoperative situation this latter assumption should never be made. By considering the way in which the mind reacts to pain, so a better judgement of pain may be reached. Psychological and social influences affect the perception of, and reaction to, pain in all individuals.

CULTURAL INFLUENCES

Response to a specific situation may be influenced by cultural background. What is wholly acceptable in one culture may be totally unacceptable in another. Traditional attitudes may determine patterns of behaviour in a society; a good example of this is a comparison of eating habits. In Western culture it is traditional to use the left hand when eating, whereas in the East, cultural influences determine that the left hand is reserved for washing after defaecation and is never used to handle food.

Pain thresholds of numerous cultural groups have been measured experimentally using various pain-inducing techniques. For example, the use of heat where a hand is placed in a bath of warm water. The temperature is raised until it becomes unbearable. At the point when the hand is withdrawn from the pain-producing stimulus the temperature is known as the pain threshold for thermal stimulus.

Such experiments have shown that the actual pain threshold of numerous cultural groups differs very little. However, the reaction to the sensation of discomfort and the tolerance of pain have shown differences between ethnic groups (Sternbach and Turskey, 1965).

In an American study of Italians, Jews and Americans of British origin, differing reactions to pain were observed in the three groups (Zborowski, 1952). The Italian patients responded to pain by complaints of discomfort caused by the pain. The Jewish patients were worried about the extent to which the pain indicated a threat to themselves, while the 'old' Americans tended to avoid complaining and minimised their pain.

The Jewish patients usually had a low tolerance of pain and described the intensity of their suffering with vivid adjectives. They believed that these intense reactions would help their pain by monopolising those around them for sympathy and assistance.

The Italians, too, showed a low pain tolerance. Crying, moaning and body gesturing are expected in their culture. However, in the presence of family and friends the Italians did not complain for fear of upsetting them. When family were present their pain was less, as they served to divert attention from it.

The 'old' Americans tended to give an efficient description of their pain. They avoided screaming and crying and only limited verbal expressions were acceptable. They also tried to maintain a sense of humour in the presence of family and were seen to withdraw and want to be alone when severe pain was present. This study presented the findings when groups were compared with each other and the descriptions mentioned were generalisations. As always, there were wide variations seen within each group.

Pain reactions often convey a great deal more than a signal that tissue damage is occurring. Different meanings can be influenced by social, cultural and environmental factors. Pain reactions can be reinforced independently of the actual physiological sensation and tissue damage. Members of cultural groups learn that some sensations are to be tolerated while others are not.

The cultural aspects of pain are indeed fascinating. Arehart-Treichel (1978) discusses an operation called trephination, performed by East African bush doctors on patients with incurable headaches. This involves scraping the patient's scalp with a large crude knife; the patient gives no evidence of feeling pain. These East African patients are quite indifferent to an operation that would almost certainly be described as painful in Western culture. Similarly, Western culture assumes that childbirth is associated with some degree of pain, whereas in some tribal populations it appears that giving birth is a totally pain-free experience for the mother, but pain is apparently experienced by the father, who labours and cries until delivery is over.

SOCIALISATION

Within any group there will be different attitudes influencing behaviour, and social conditioning will determine the ways people react to life events. Imagine a crowded shopping centre on a Saturday afternoon; a three year old falls and hurts his knee and cries. In such a circumstance the reaction of one parent might be to comfort the child while another may display anger, or even punish the child for falling over. Such attitudes in the growing years help to define and condition reactions to pain in later years.

SEX

Western culture has different attitudes to boys and girls. In their early years boys are encouraged to be 'brave', while it is more acceptable for girls to be emotional and demonstrative about hurt; bravery is largely a male concept carried into adult life. It appears that this traditional view about pain may cause undue suffering in male surgical patients. Studies have shown that nurses administer less analgesia to male patients than to female patients (Bond, 1979). The assumption drawn from these findings is that hospital personnel expect men to have less pain and that the men reported less pain, probably deriving from the cultural and social characteristics of their upbringing.

PERSONALITY

A variety of personality traits have been associated with differences in the reaction to pain but the results of various studies are conflicting. However, the attitude of a person to pain will be determined to some extent by individual personality. There is evidence that a higher pain tolerance may be related to extroversion as measured in personality tests (Boyle and Parbrook, 1977). These tests may take the form of a questionnaire in which the patient has to answer yes or no to a series of questions related to psychological features. The questions determine emotional stability, extroversion, tendency to psychotic traits and tendency to exaggerate. The Eysenck Personality Inventory measures two dimensions of personality regarded as fundamental because they are related directly to the physiological activity of the central nervous system. The dimensions are stability/neuroticism and introversion/extroversion. It appears that people who are found to be emotional and sociable are those who complain of pain and receive more medication. Less sociable and emotional people still feel pain but tend not to complain about it. Those with an introverted personality appear to feel pain sooner and more intensely than others, but complain less (Bond, 1979).

Janis (1958) studied a small group of patients pre-operatively and concluded that people awaiting surgery may be divided into three personality groups in respect of their attitudes to operations. The first tends to be panic-stricken and shrinks from surgery; when faced with the event they cope badly and demand and seek attention. The second group shows little or no fear, are relaxed, calm and confident that all will be well. They minimise the danger to themselves and display an avoidance-coping response. These people generally recover well after their operation, but if faced with complications they find the set-back difficult to cope with emotionally, probably because they had denied that a complication was possible. The third group are moderately fearful but not overwhelmed by their feelings. They may be eager to obtain facts about treatment and tend to build up a framework upon which to develop their emotional safeguards in advance. The nurse's recognition of personality factors is an important part of pre-operative assessment (see p. 17).

EMOTIONAL INFLUENCES

Anxiety

Illness, especially if severe, or of uncertain outcome, inevitably raises levels of anxiety. Anxiety may be experienced and manifested by individuals in many different ways according to the psychological background and physical make-up of each. There are many possible combinations of the physiological and psychological signs of anxiety.

Detection of anxiety requires that the nurse is able to recognise some of the suggestive signs or behaviour patterns associated with it:

Heart rate increased 10 beats or more over 'basic' rate for that patient.
Systolic blood pressure increased 10mmHg over 'basic' pressure.
Dryness of mouth.

Inability or unwillingness to look at nurse while speaking.
Rapid or darting eye movements.
Perspiration.
Generalised trembling or shivering or tremor of hands.
Overactivity or unusual restlessness.
Clenching of fists.
Nail biting or lip biting.
Expression of fears verbally and specifically.
Irrelevant conversation – keeps changing subject.
Very rapid speech, abruptness, interruption.
Constant conversation, must be interrupted for next point.
Irritability or general impatience.
Description of tension or inability to relax.
Expressions of great self-sufficiency, or denial of the seriousness of
    illness or surgery.
Making no attempt to seek any information from the nurse when
    the opportunity is present.
Taut or strained facial expression.
Facial, arm or shoulder tics.
Marked pallor or flushing of the face.
Rigid or protective posture, with arms folded across chest or hands
    in front of parts of face, e.g. mouth during visit.
Hesitation before answering, stammering, difficulty concentrating
    or remembering simple questions or statements, repetitive
    statements.
Crying, or evidence of crying before visit.

Acute pain provokes anxiety, and anxiety heightens pain; many of
the expressions of anxiety listed above are also seen as expressions of
pain. The emotional responses to both feelings may be very similar
and are frequently interrelated. Nurses need to be able to distinguish
'the chicken from the egg'. If anxiety is increasing pain, then the
cause of the anxiety should be sought and dealt with, if on the other
hand the pain is causing anxiety, then relief of that pain will lessen
this reaction to it (Fig. 1/1).

Relief
While the emotion of anxiety serves to heighten pain, that of relief
does much to decrease what is felt. Beecher (1956) compared the
analgesic needs of soldiers with those of civilians with similar injuries
and found that the soldiers required fewer pain-killers. The civilians

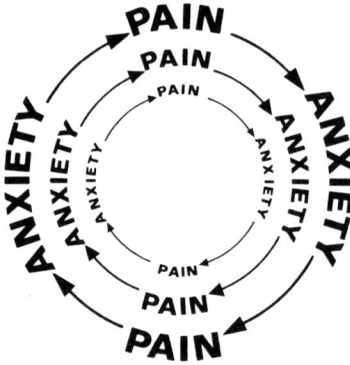

Fig. 1/1 The vicious circle of pain and anxiety

had found themselves, through their injuries, to be in an unexpectedly frightening and possibly life-threatening situation, whereas the soldiers, having been wounded, were relieved of the possibility of dying and had escaped from the terror of the battlefield.

Distraction
A decrease in the pain experienced may be brought about by distraction. An example of this is seen in sportsmen who frequently receive severe injury during the course of a game but do not become aware of the resulting pain until the match is over. The excitement and distraction of the game draw attention away from the injury (see p. 147).

Previous experience
People who have had unpleasant experiences in their lives tend to remember them. Most of us can bring to mind an occasion which produced discomfort in childhood, perhaps the death of a relative, or an accident to ourselves.

The experience of severe pain is easily recalled: if such an episode was not understood, or was managed in a way which appeared harsh or inadequate, then the prospect of a painful episode is likely to increase anxiety. Such experiences of unrelieved pain have caused some patients to smuggle their own analgesics into hospital (Tight Fisted Analgesia) (*Lancet*, 1976).

REFERENCES

Arehart-Treichel, J. (1978). The great pain plan. *Science News*, **114**, 266–7.

Beecher, H. K. (1956) Relationship of significance of wound to the pain experienced. *Journal of the American Medical Association*, **161**, 1609–13.

Bond, M. R. (1979). *Pain: Its Nature, Analysis and Treatment*. Churchill Livingstone, Edinburgh.

Boyle, P. and Parbrook, G. D. (1977). The interrelation of personality and postoperative factors. *British Journal of Anaesthesia*, **49**, 259.

Editorial (1976). Tight fisted analgesia. *Lancet*, **1**, 1338.

Janis, I. L. (1958). *Psychological Stress*. John Wiley and Sons, New York.

Sternbach, R. A. and Turskey, B. (1965). Ethnic differences among housewives in psychophysical and skin potential responses to electric shock. *Psychophysiology*, **1**, 241–6.

Zborowski, M. (1952). Cultural component in response to pain. *Journal of Social Issues*, 16–30.

Chapter Two

INTRODUCING NEUROANATOMY

The human nervous system consists of three parts:

1. The central nervous system
2. The peripheral nervous system
3. The autonomic nervous system.

All three parts are intimately connected and their effects are inter-related.

THE CENTRAL NERVOUS SYSTEM

This consists of the brain and the spinal cord. The brain lies within the skull and is continuous with the spinal cord through a large opening in the base of the skull, the foramen magnum. The spinal cord passes down the vertebral canal which is a tube-shaped space within the bony spine (Fig. 2/1).

The brain (Fig. 2/2)
The brain includes the two hemispheres, right and left (the cerebrum), the brainstem and the cerebellum. Each hemisphere is divided into four lobes, the frontal, parietal, temporal and occipital. Although the functions of the brain are highly integrated certain regions have specific functions: the frontal lobes are concerned with some aspects of behaviour, emotion and motor function; the parietal lobes are associated with bodily sensations; the temporal lobes are associated with the sensations of taste, smell and hearing; and the occipital lobes are concerned with vision (Fig. 2/3). Speech is localised in the dominant hemisphere which in right-handed people is the left. In

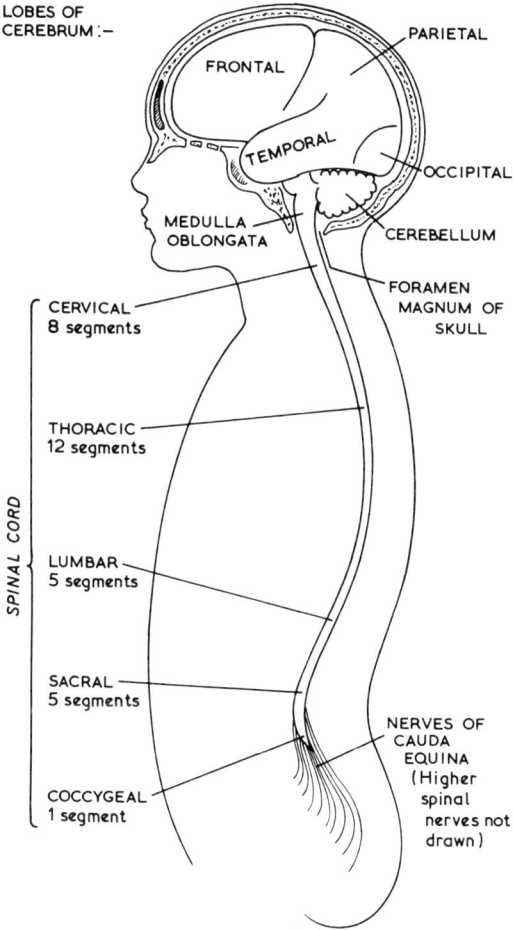

LOBES OF
CEREBRUM :—

FRONTAL

PARIETAL

TEMPORAL

OCCIPITAL

MEDULLA
OBLONGATA

CEREBELLUM

FORAMEN OF
MAGNUM OF
SKULL

CERVICAL
8 segments

THORACIC
12 segments

SPINAL CORD

LUMBAR
5 segments

SACRAL
5 segments

NERVES OF
CAUDA
EQUINA
(Higher
spinal
nerves not
drawn)

COCCYGEAL
1 segment

Fig. 2/1   The central nervous system

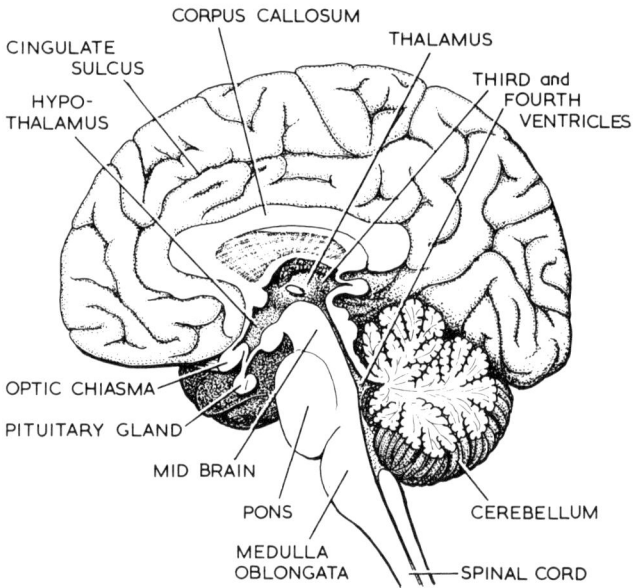

Fig. 2/2   A lateral view through the mid-line of the brain to show the relationship of the cerebral hemisphere, brainstem and spinal cord

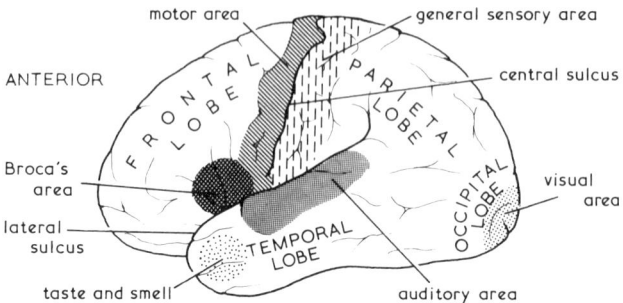

Fig. 2/3   Lateral view of the lobes of the hemisphere showing the main areas of function

those who are left-handed the speech centre is poorly localised in the right hemisphere.

The brainstem lies below the cerebral hemispheres and is a direct upward extension of the spinal cord into the base of the brain within the skull. The upper portion of the brainstem is called the mid-brain and contains the important co-ordinating area of the central nervous system known as the reticular formation. The mid-brain also contains the nuclei of some of the cranial nerves. Below the mid-brain lies the pons which also contains some nuclei of the cranial nerves as well as motor fibres descending from higher in the brain and sensory fibres travelling upwards to higher portions of the brain. The pons also contains fibres associated with the cerebellum which is a large structure at the same level as the pons, resting in the angle between the spinal cord and the occipital lobes. The cerebellum is concerned with balance and the co-ordination of movement.

The lowest part of the brainstem is called the medulla oblongata (Fig. 2/2) and also contains cranial nerve nuclei. The vital centres which control essential functions such as heart beat and respiration are located in this area as well.

The spinal cord

The spinal cord starts at the level of the foramen magnum which is the largest opening in the base of the skull, and runs down to the level of the second lumbar vertebra. As said earlier the cord lies in the middle of the bony channel within the vertebrae called the spinal canal. Twelve pairs of cranial nerves arise from the brainstem and, similarly, 31 pairs of spinal nerve roots arise from the spinal cord. They each emerge laterally from the cord to form mixed spinal nerves, that is, they contain both sensory and motor nerves. As these spinal nerves emerge from the vertebral canal they may divide and rejoin several times as they distribute themselves throughout the body in the peripheral nervous system.

THE PERIPHERAL NERVOUS SYSTEM

This consists of the spinal nerves which travel to and from the spinal cord, and the facial nerves which travel to and from the brainstem. Some peripheral nerves contain only sensory fibres which carry information from the body to the central nervous system, while others are purely motor-carrying impulses from the central nervous system to the head and body. The majority of peripheral nerves are, however, mixed, and contain both motor and sensory fibres.

The nerve fibres within the peripheral nervous system can be classified into three main groups. 'A' fibres have a large diameter, being up to 20 micrometres thick, and have a myelin sheath around them. 'B' fibres are also myelinated, but are smaller being less than 3 micrometres thick. The smallest fibres are called 'C' fibres and are up to 1 micrometre thick and not myelinated. These three groups are not distinct and merge into each other. The myelin sheath is made up of alternate layers of lecithin and protein and gets thinner as the nerve fibres themselves get thinner. Nerve fibres are able to conduct electrical impulses down their length. The impulses travel fastest down the larger diameter nerves, and the presence of a myelin sheath around the nerve fibre also improves its speed of transmission (see Figs. 2/4, 2/5).

THE AUTONOMIC NERVOUS SYSTEM

This consists of the sympathetic and parasympathetic nervous systems; in general terms these two parts have opposing actions and the final effect is due to the interplay of their opposing actions.

The autonomic nervous system acts more or less automatically: there is no voluntary control. The autonomic system controls the size of the pupil of the eye; the secretion of glands such as the salivary and lacrimal; and the activity of smooth muscle in blood vessels, the bladder and various organs of the gastro-intestinal tract.

After leaving the brainstem and the spinal cord, autonomic nerves connect with neurones which lie in discrete collections of nerve cells, fibres and synapses called ganglia. Nerve fibres pass from these ganglia to their final destinations. These autonomic ganglia are situated parallel to the vertebral column or, in some instances, on cranial nerves.

The actions of the *sympathetic nervous system* are largely mediated by the transmitters adrenaline and noradrenaline which are released from the nerve endings to act on peripheral structures where they may cause blood vessels to constrict, the pupil to dilate and the heart rate to increase.

The *parasympathetic nervous system* releases acetylcholine at its nerve terminals; this causes the pupil to constrict, the heart rate to decrease and a variety of effects in the intestines and bladder.

To sum up, the parasympathetic system controls the routine

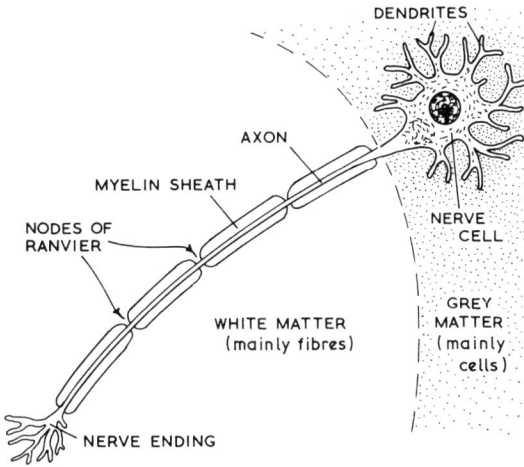

Fig. 2/4   The structure of a neurone

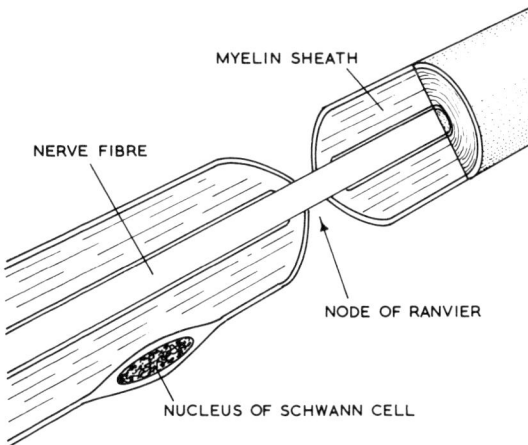

Fig. 2/5   A longitudinal section through a myelinated
nerve fibre

maintenance functions of the body, while the sympathetic system prepares the body for action – the 'fight or flight' reaction. The autonomic nervous system also has certain sensory functions, and may carry pain impulses from blood vessels and viscera.

NERVOUS TISSUE (Figs. 2/4, 2/5)

Nervous tissue consists of nerve cells, nerve fibres and the surrounding supportive tissue, glia. Each nerve cell has several extensions, or arms, sticking out around itself. One of these is larger than the rest and is named the nerve fibre. The cell and the fibre together constitute a single neurone. Nerve fibres with similar functions tend to run together in pathways or tracts in the central nervous system.

Most nerve fibres are covered by a fatty white layer, myelin. Where there are large collections of nerve fibres together, their myelin sheaths make the tissue look pale so that it is called *white matter*. Those areas which contain large collections of nerve cells together or nerve fibres without myelin sheaths look dark and are called *grey matter*. Grey matter is found in the central portions of the spinal cord, the surface layer of the cerebral cortex, the basal ganglia and some of the brainstem nuclei; elsewhere it is mostly white matter.

Chapter Three

PAIN PATHWAYS

The sensation known as pain is commonly applied to descriptions of any unpleasant experiences, for example, memories and emotions. Much debate has gone into the present medical definition of pain being an 'unpleasant sensation usually associated with tissue damage and which may be described in terms of tissue damage' (Merskey et al, 1979). Such debate was necessary because pain is a major cause of suffering and a tight definition enables doctors, nurses and researchers to concentrate their respective efforts in the most efficient manner. Postoperative pain is due to tissue damage resulting from the pathological condition; the surgery used to correct it; or the complications resulting from either.

RECEPTORS

In skin, muscle, viscera and around bones are microscopic organs called *receptors* which, when stimulated, are capable of exciting their associated nerves. The term *receptor* means a tiny organ which receives stimuli and converts the stimulus energy into electrical energy, which triggers a nerve to fire. There are various kinds of receptors in the body, most of which respond best to a particular stimulus, such as vibration, touch, or hot and cold.

Pain receptors (Fig. 3/1)
Pain may be produced by the over-stimulation of receptors capable of responding to a variety of normal stimuli. These are called polymodal receptors and usually respond to mechanical injury, chemical stimulation or thermal irritation. The other major group of receptors

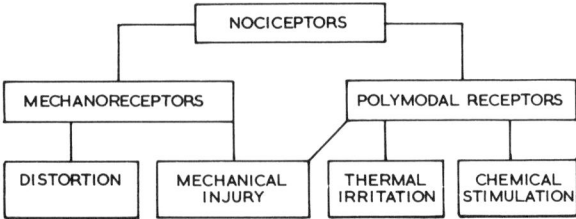

Fig. 3/1   A classification of pain receptors

associated with pain are structurally simple, resembling bare nerve endings. They respond normally to mechanical injury or distortion.

Strong mechanical stimulation, such as pinching, and strong thermal stimulation by very hot or cold sensations will give rise to painful sensations. The chemical irritants which commonly cause pain include potassium ions which leak out of damaged cells, hydrogen ions which collect around infected tissues or where tissues are not supplied with sufficient oxygen. Bradykinin and serotonin are both chemical 'messengers' known to stimulate pain receptors and are released into damaged tissues. A chemical, prostaglandin, may be released into inflamed tissues, making the receptors in those tissues more sensitive to painful stimuli. Prostaglandin is important since many of the aspirin-like analgesics act by inhibiting the production of it.

How a receptor works
Each receptor is connected to a nerve and when the receptor is stimulated, it excites the nerve into firing an electrical impulse down its length (Fig. 3/2).

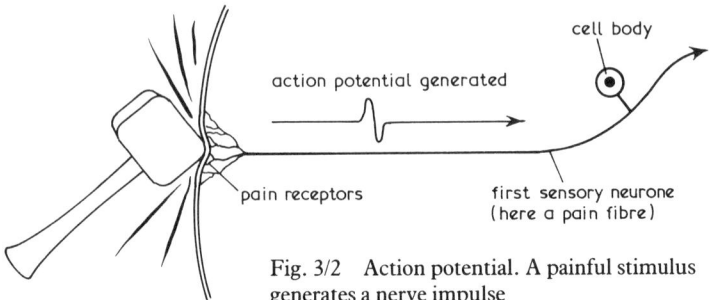

Fig. 3/2   Action potential. A painful stimulus generates a nerve impulse

Classification of nerves

Nerves have been classified according to thickness and whether or not there is a layer of fatty myelin insulation around them (Fig. 3/3). Nerves with the largest diameter conduct impulses faster than the

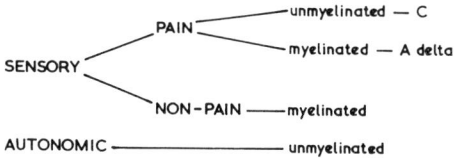

Fig. 3/3 A classification of nerves

smaller nerves, and the presence of a myelin sheath around the nerves allows them to conduct impulses even faster (see p.26).

Nerves may thus be classified according to their size:

1. The largest, myelinated fibres conduct impulses from the brain to muscles, making them contract.
2. Medium-sized nerves with myelin sheaths conduct non-painful sensory information.
3. Smallest diameter nerves, with or without myelin sheaths, carry pain impulses. These travel more slowly than any other sensory or motor impulses.

PAIN IMPULSES

The fibres carrying pain impulses to the brain may belong either to the sensory nervous system or the autonomic system. The autonomic nerves are unmyelinated fibres which conduct impulses of which we are normally unaware.

Pain impulses which are transmitted in autonomic nerves may originate in viscera or blood vessel walls and may have to travel some distance in the body before crossing over to the pain-conducting fibres of the sensory nervous system. The sensory fibres form nerves, some of which are purely sensory; the majority, however, are mixed, having both motor and sensory fibres. Nerves may be visible to the naked eye at operation (Fig. 3/4). From their origins nerves progress towards the spinal cord, joining together to form plexuses such as the brachial and sacral. Within the spinal canal, the large nerves divide into a motor section which emerges anteriorly from the spinal cord,

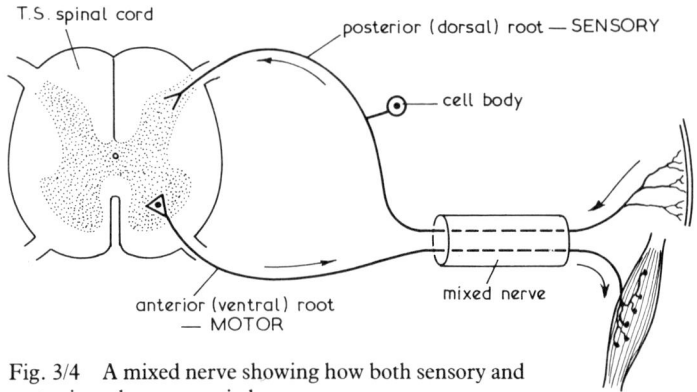

Fig. 3/4   A mixed nerve showing how both sensory and motor impulses are carried

and a sensory root, which enters the posterior or dorsal aspect of the spinal cord. The sensory fibres pass to the relevant area of the cord depending on the sensations carried (Fig. 3/5).

Synapses (Fig. 3/6)
Nerves are linked together so that the electrical impulses travelling along one nerve may be transmitted to near-by nerves. These electrical junctions are called synapses; they will conduct electrical impulses in one direction only because they work by releasing chemicals called

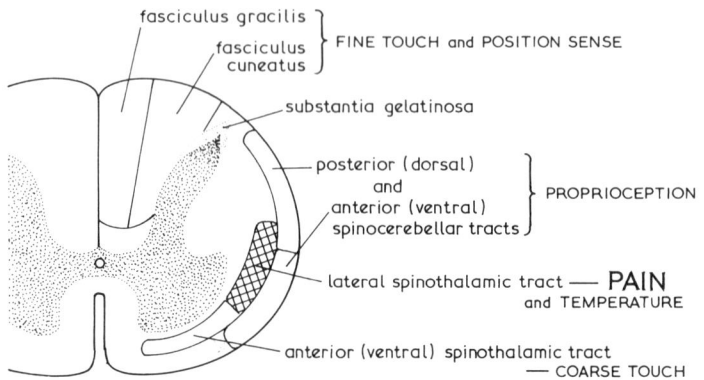

Fig. 3/5   A cross-section of the spinal cord showing sensory tracts

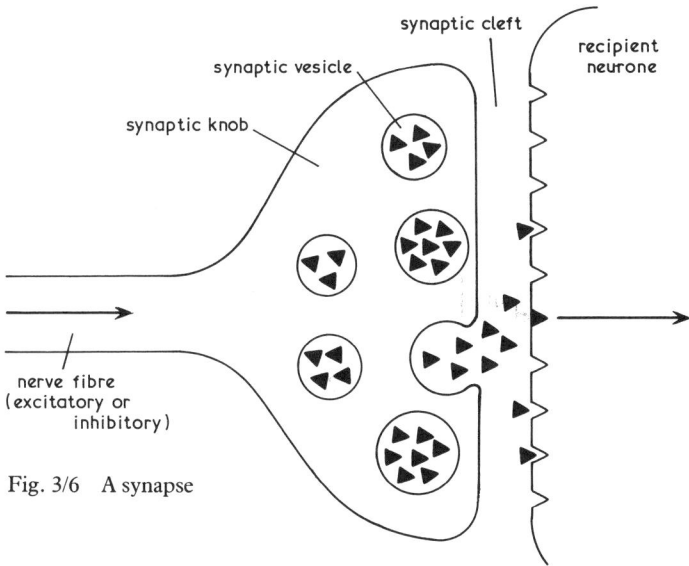

Fig. 3/6   A synapse

transmitters from the end of one of the nerves to be received by chemical receptors in the adjacent nerve.

Transmitters
There are different kinds of transmitter chemicals, each of which will be picked up only by its own type of receptor. Some transmitters will cause their receptors to generate electrical impulses in the secondary nerves, and thus the original impulse may be propagated onward. Alternatively, some transmitters may cause their receptors to make the secondary nerves less electrically excitable, thus inhibiting the propagation of the original electrical impulse. Each nerve may make several synapses with its surrounding nerves and in turn may have several nerves' synapses on itself. The electrical state of any particular nerve will depend upon the interplay of the excitatory and inhibitory transmitters released on to it at any given moment (Fig. 3/7).

Pain-gates (Fig. 3/8)
Each pain-conducting fibre terminates within the dorsal horn by linking with a secondary nerve fibre. Some first-order pain-conducting fibres may link with several of these second-order fibres. Some of

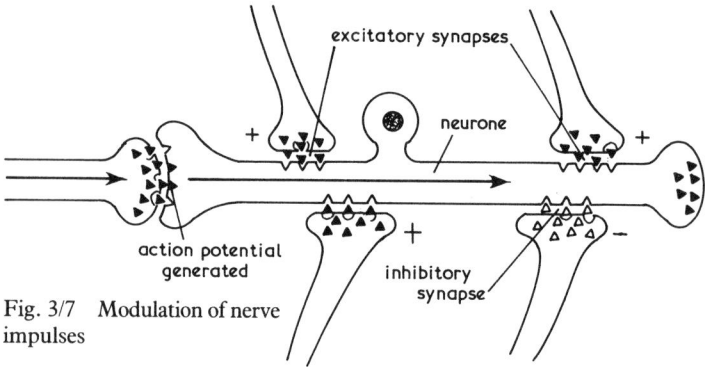

Fig. 3/7 Modulation of nerve impulses

them may also form cross-links with other fibres in the dorsal horn which, rather than simply conduct the pain impulses upward to the brain, may serve to modify those impulses. These modifying fibres in the spinal cord have been described as 'pain-gates'. They may completely inhibit the passage of painful impulses (Fig. 3/8) or they may amplify them and make the final pain felt, worse.

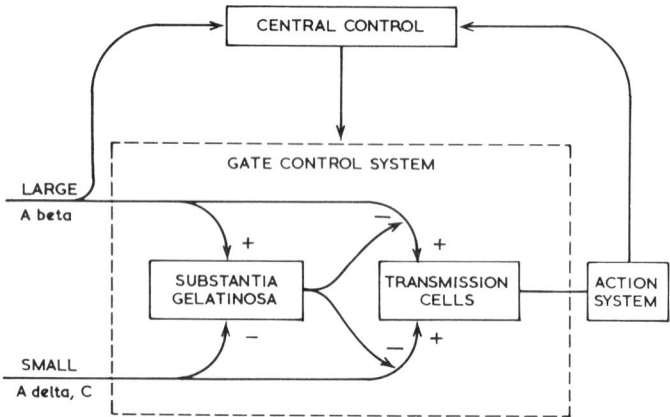

Fig. 3/8 Pain gate. The substantia gelatinosa cells may inhibit the passage of impulses from the large and small sensory fibres coming into the spinal cord, as they cross over to the transmission cells which will take the impulses up the cord for further action

When the body is subjected to a painful stimulus, the pain receptors will be stimulated and will trigger their attached, fine diameter, slow-conducting nerves to fire impulses centrally, towards the spinal cord. However, stimuli which are strong enough to trigger the pain receptors will also be strong enough to stimulate near-by non-pain receptors. These non-pain receptors will also trigger their associated nerves to fire. Because non-painful sensation travels in wider diameter nerves than pain, these wider diameter fibres conduct their non-painful impulses to the spinal cord faster than the pain impulses, and arrive first. In the dorsal horn of the spinal cord, it appears that these non-painful impulses are able to close the pain-gates before the pain impulses reach them. In this way, the pain may appear much reduced, or even absent. These inhibitory pain-gates have been utilised in the treatment of both chronic and acute pain. By stimulating nerves coming from a painful region with strong, but non-painful, stimuli, such as heat, vibration or an electrical buzzing sensation (TNS, see p. 148), the apparent pain felt by the patient is often reduced. However, if the pain impulses persist and are strong enough, they may re-open the pain-gates, allowing free passage of the pain impulses through the dorsal horn and on to higher parts of the nervous system.

The pain-gates in the spinal cord may be controlled by impulses travelling down the cord from the brain itself. These descending impulses may account for the pain-numbing effects of distraction, or the pain-enhancing effects of emotion. Years of social conditioning may pre-set the level of inhibitory tone in this descending pathway, while the effects of drugs or disease may also temporarily change it. Both antidepressant drugs and opiates may relieve pain by stimulating the descending pain inhibitory pathway. Opiates may also directly affect the pain-gates in the spinal cord, closing them by mimicking naturally occurring transmitters.

Anterolateral tracts

After passing through the pain-gates of the dorsal horn, pain impulses travelling along their second-order neurones mostly cross over to the opposite side of the spinal cord within a few segments of the one in which they first entered the cord. They then collect into a discrete bundle of fibres, all carrying pain information upward to the brain, and called the anterolateral tract (Fig. 3/9). A small proportion of these second-order fibres travel to the anterolateral tract of the same side, without crossing over until they have reached the lowest portions

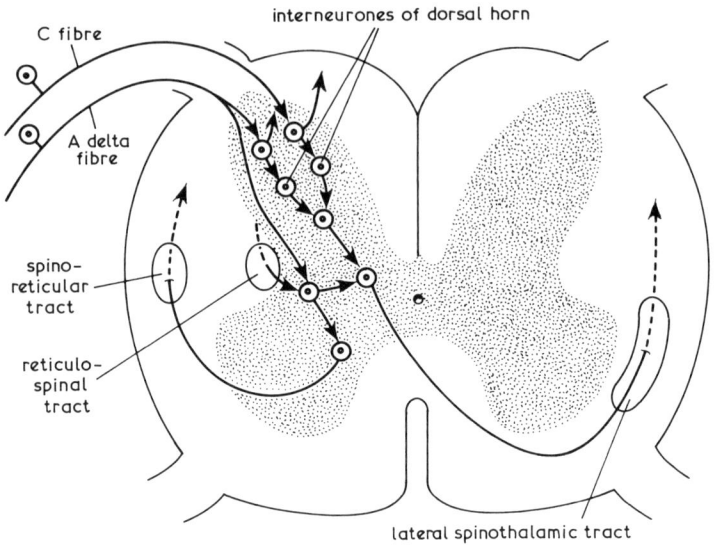

C fibre

A delta
fibre

interneurones of dorsal horn

spino-
reticular
tract

reticulo-
spinal
tract

lateral spinothalamic tract

Fig. 3/9   Cross-section of the
spinal cord showing how pain
fibres enter, cross over and then
ascend

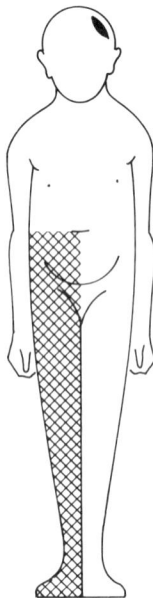

Fig. 3/10   A lesion affecting
the sensory cortex on one side
of the brain will cause sensory
changes on the opposite side

of the brain itself. All the sensory fibres travelling from the body to the brain cross over to the opposite side of the brain eventually, so that all sensation, including pain, from the right side of the body, travels to the left side of the brain and vice versa.

Sensations, including pain, coming from the *face*, however, travel in the facial nerve. Impulses coming from the face do *not* cross over to the opposite side of the brain. If a patient has a tumour or lesion of the brain causing sensory symptoms in the *body*, the symptoms will be on the opposite side of the body to the side of the brain affected by the lesion (Fig. 3/10). If the same tumour causes sensory symptoms in the face, they would be on the same side as the tumour.

The anterolateral tracts each contain two main bundles of pain-carrying fibres, the spinothalamic and spinoreticular tracts. Their names simply refer to where they originated – the spine, and their destinations – the thalamus and the reticular formation respectively.

Spinothalamic tract (Fig. 3/11)

This is the simpler and more laterally placed of the two tracts. It largely carries information about the position and quality of the pain. The tract contains bundles of long nerve fibres, each of which originates in the spinal cord near to where its primary nerve fibre entered. While most of these fibres end in the lower, lateral parts of the thalamus, where they synapse with their third-order neurones, some fibres of each side branch off to a small area called the medial geniculate body, where they meet and synapse with their own third-order neurones. All the third-order neurones from the spinothalamic pathway continue upward to the cortex (the outermost layer of the brain), where there is a region reserved for sensation of all kinds. The whole of each side of the body is represented on the sensory cortex of the opposite side, together with facial sensation coming from the same side (Fig. 3/12).

Spinoreticular tract (Fig. 3/13)

This pathway is the more medial of the two. After ascending the spinal cord almost all of its fibres enter and synapse in the region of the brain called the reticular formation. This area is full of synapses, with nerves travelling to all parts of the brain. The third-order neurones from the spinoreticular pathway may therefore be distributed to many regions of the brain. Some go to the areas associated with emotional responses to pain – the limbic system, while others may travel to regions which control hormonal responses to sensations,

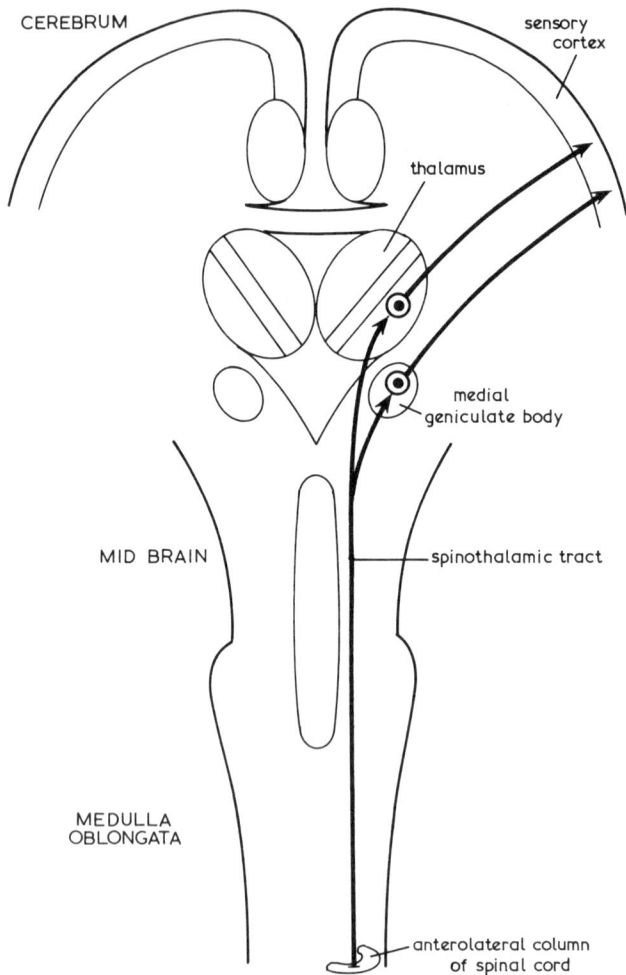

Fig. 3/11   The spinothalamic tract

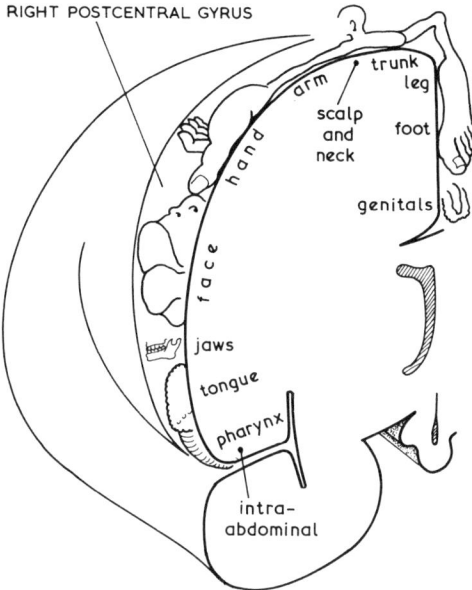

Fig. 3/12   The sensory cortex. A cross-section of
the human brain showing the cortical representation
of bodily sensation

such as the hypothalamus. There are fibres which run upward and
forward to the frontal lobes, where past experiences may be stored,
and comparisons with the present stimulus made.

Inhibitory pathway (Fig. 3/14)
A descending inhibitory pathway, which has the ability to control
painful impulses as they enter the spinal cord, has been mentioned
(p. 35). This pathway appears to start in the lower lateral portions of
the thalamus, where fibres of the spinothalamic pathway are synapsing.
It then passes downward to the reticular formation, through which it
travels, synapsing on its way with the fibres of the spinoreticular
pathway. The inhibitory pathway then goes down the spinal cord,
travelling in the middle of the dorsal horn and synapsing with
incoming sensory fibres carrying pain impulses.

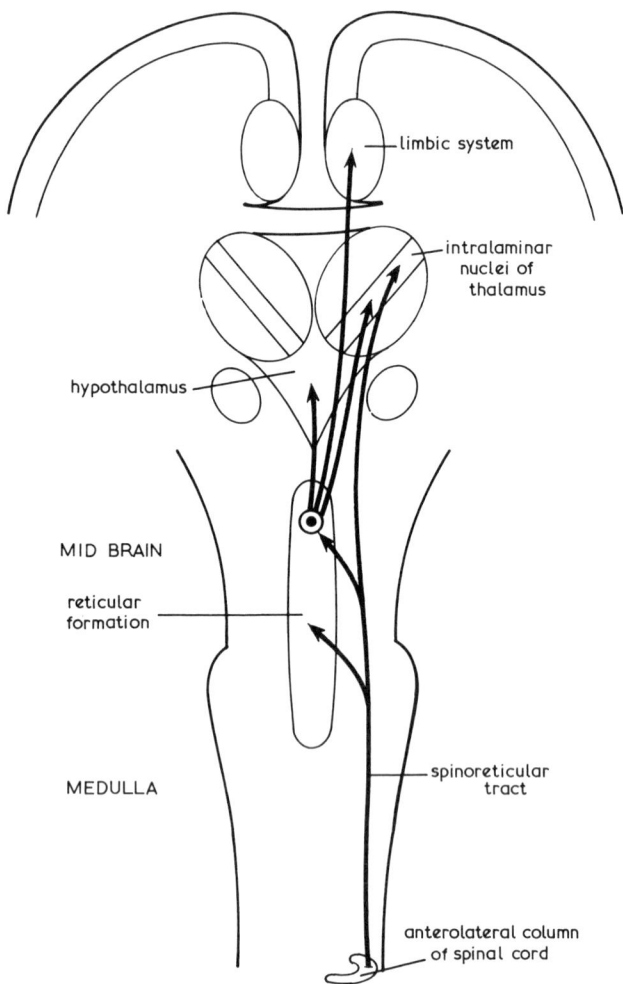

Fig. 3/13   The spinorecticular tract

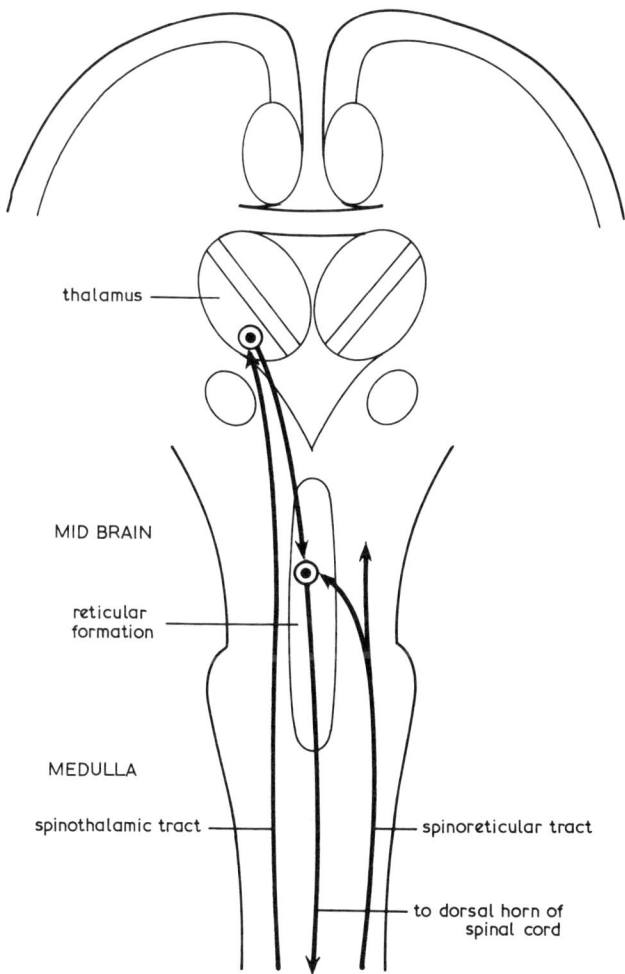

thalamus

MID BRAIN

reticular
formation

MEDULLA

spinothalamic tract

spinoreticular tract

to dorsal horn of
spinal cord

Fig. 3/14   The descending inhibitory pathway

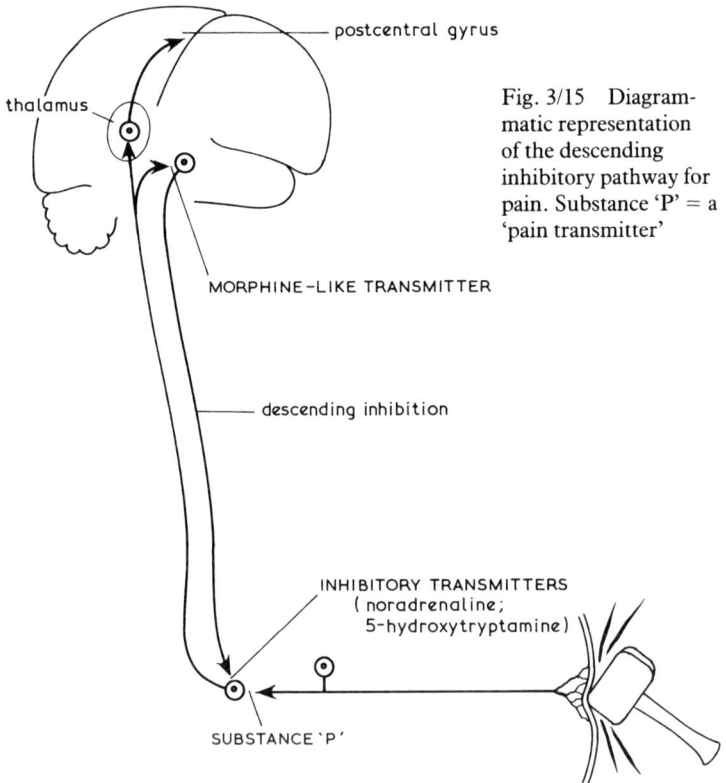

Fig. 3/15 Diagrammatic representation of the descending inhibitory pathway for pain. Substance 'P' = a 'pain transmitter'

Modifying painful sensations (Fig. 3/15)

The intensity of a painful sensation can be modified in the spinal cord and, at a higher level, in the brain. Most of the changes are carried out without conscious effort or control, despite the fact that reducing pain in this way is an active process involving the activation of inhibitory pathways and the release of inhibitory chemical transmitters. The responses to pain may be graded according to the intensity of the stimuli and the amount of inhibition used against them. If a hot stone were put into the hand, it would be dropped without thinking. However, if a hot and valuable plate were put into the hand, the person would juggle with it or hold it long enough to put it down without breaking. The reflex dropping action used with the hot stone would have been suppressed and replaced with much more complex behaviour, controlled this time by the brain. In so doing, the pain which was being perceived almost instantly with the hot stone, may be suppressed long enough in the case of the valuable plate to enable it to be put down safely.

REFERENCE

Merskey, H. et al (1979). Pain terms: a list with definitions and usage 1979. *Pain*, **79,** 6, 249.

BIBLIOGRAPHY

Wall, P. D. (1984). The challenge of pain. *The Listener*, 26 July, pp. 7–8.

Chapter Four

ASSESSMENT OF PAIN

Accurate estimation of pain and its effects is not a simple task. It demands time and understanding and requires skills of observation and communication.

Any attempt to evaluate pain must begin with the recognition that pain is a subjective phenomenon, and that many factors influence its perception, response and reporting. It is these phenomena which may cause problems both for the assessor and the person experiencing the pain.

Nurses should remind themselves that they may hold pre-conceived ideas, or even misconceptions, about pain which may make accurate assessment very difficult. The person in pain also has attitudes about how pain should be reported and reacted to. The attitudes of both the nurse and the patient are shaped by their social and cultural backgrounds as well as by personality characteristics (see Chapter 1).

Wherever possible the assessment of pain must be achieved with the patient. To do this effectively, both patient and nurse should be as comfortable and relaxed as possible, the nurse sitting, or standing near to the patient on the same level so that eye contact is easy (see Fig. 5/2 p. 62).

ASSESSMENT

A pain assessment may take place in all sorts of circumstances and surroundings. The nurse has to judge which questions are relevant in each particular situation where there might be a need to make an assessment. It would be inhumane to take half an hour to assess severe, acute pain which is obviously getting worse while detailed questions are being asked. In such a case suitable pain-relief should be given after preliminary enquiry, the details coming later when the patient is able to communicate without experiencing extreme discomfort.

Before asking questions relating to pain the nurse should establish the patient's ability to communicate. In some cases verbal communication is lost, or seriously impaired (for example, in patients who have suffered head injury or who are mentally handicapped) so that information cannot be obtained through conversation. When this is the case, observation of physiological signs and behavioural changes can give clues to the presence and severity of pain. Family members or others close to the patient can usually provide helpful information about reactions and responses to unpleasant stimuli.

Perhaps the most important aspect of assessing pain in any circumstance is listening. When the patient is encouraged to talk, the listening nurse can become aware of the nature of the pain on a physical level and of its implications for that individual, taking into account the cultural background, past experiences and current anxieties. Talking about pain or discomfort affords the nurse the opportunity to convey reassurance by letting the patient know that she cares and is interested in him. Talking in this way means that nurses should not tell the patients about pain but rather let the patients tell them. This is possible when the conversation pays attention not only to details about physical pain but also to the various symptoms associated with it. Many of the accompanying problems can be relieved by nursing measures which can only be appropriately planned after first obtaining as much relevant information as possible through communication and observation with the patient and the relatives.

TAKING A PAIN HISTORY WITH THE PRE-OPERATIVE PATIENT

Frequently surgery is planned because the patient has a painful condition which requires radical treatment to remove or prevent the cause of the pain – gallstones are an obvious example. However, surgery may also be performed for conditions which were not manifest by pain, for example thyroidectomy.

Pre-operative assessment of any pain that the patient has suffered, whether or not related to the reason for surgery, will be of value in planning the postoperative nursing care with respect to pain relief.

Knowing how a patient reacted to pain in a given situation in the past should give the nurse some insight into the likely response to discomfort encountered while in hospital. It will also allow the patient an opportunity to express any particular reactions, fears or unpleasant memories about previous painful experiences.

Assuming that the patient is able to communicate, there are four main areas which the surgical nurse can explore when making an assessment of pain.

1. How is the pain?

Many people readily define and describe their pain. They can tell you what type of pain they are experiencing, or have experienced, by using descriptive words to paint a picture. Adjectives such as burning, aching and gripping may be used by the sufferer. However, when the patient seems unsure of how to describe the type of pain and can't think of suitable words, then the nurse might offer a list to pick from: 'Is your pain dull, aching or throbbing?'

Sometimes the nurse may have to use terms other than 'pain' to help patients make their description – the terms 'discomfort' or 'feeling' may better fit the patient's perception of what is happening. As well as having a description of the type of pain, one needs to know how severe it is. Again, the nurse can offer words for the patient to choose from, 'Is the pain mild or slight, moderate or severe?' A visual chart can be helpful in assessing the severity of the pain being experienced and from such a chart a rating scale can be obtained (Fig. 4/1). This gives the patient's estimate of pain being experienced at any one time and, if repeated over a period, can be used to

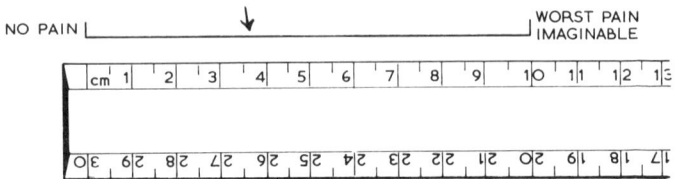

Fig. 4/1 Visual analogue for assessment of severity of pain. The patient is asked to mark the 10cm line on the point between the two extremes where he estimates his pain to be. A measurement can then be made of this subjective assessment

compare with ratings at different times and following pain-relieving methods. Used in this way, pain-assessment charts can become aids to evaluation (Fig. 4/2).

2. When is the pain?

The occurrence of pain may or may not be related to specific events. It is important to know when the pain first occurred, how long it has been present, or how long it lasted during intermittent episodes. The duration of episodes of pain may be fairly consistent, or the duration of pain may alter. Enquiry should be made about possible relationships with other events: perhaps the pain is related to eating, walking or resting. Ask if, when the pain is present, the patient is able to do anything to alter its duration.

3. Where is the pain?

The patient should be asked where the pain is. Sometimes it is easier to ask him to show you where he feels the discomfort. Ask if there is pain only in one place or whether more than one area is affected. When this is the case it should be established whether the pains from the different areas feel the same or are different from each other. Pain may not be identified in a specific area, so ask if it seems to move.

Discomfort may be felt as deep or superficial pain. Some patients may be very clear about where they think the pain is coming from and therefore suspect a cause. Alternatively, anxiety might be expressed because no obvious reason for the pain exists and the patient is at a loss to understand why he should be suffering.

4. Effects of the pain

Patients should be asked about the effect that the pain has on them. Chronic pain and acute pain usually bring forth very different reactions. Enquiry about the patient's perception of his pain and the response to it can be made. Some may accept and tolerate pain, remaining calm and controlled, while others admit to distress and show these feelings. Pain, especially when prolonged or chronic, may cause resentment and depression, whereas anxiety and fear frequently accompany acute pain. The pain may be interfering with many aspects of the patient's normal life, so ask about sleep and social activity, work and relationships with others.

Examples of pre-operative assessment of pain and patients' reactions
Mr Brown is a booked admission who has proven gallstones and has

PAIN ASSESSMENT CHART

NAME Susan Jones   Time 14.00   Date 3.6.84   Ward K

OPERATION/DIAGNOSIS Above knee amputation (12.5.84)   Hospital No. AA 1234

AVERAGE Pain Level
in past 24 hours

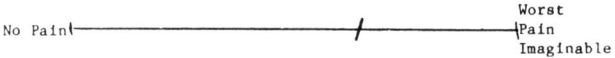

```
                                                              Worst
No Pain ─────────────────────────────────── / ──────────────┤Pain
                                                              Imaginable
```
....

WORST Pain Experienced
in past 24 hours

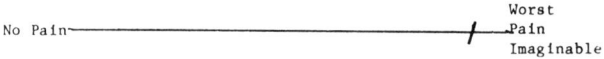

```
                                                              Worst
No Pain ───────────────────────────────────────────── / ─────Pain
                                                              Imaginable
```
....

PAIN NOW

```
                                                              Worst
No Pain ───────────── / ──────────────────────────────────── Pain
                                                              Imaginable
```
....

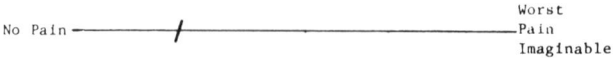

AVERAGE SCORE: 6.5   WORST SCORE: 9.1   PRESENT SCORE: 2.4

Drugs :- 30mg MST Continus 08.00 and 22.00
         Pethidine 100mg stat pre dressing 11.00
         Dihydrocodeine 30mg prn last given 12.00
....

Fig. 4/2   Pain assessment chart

come into hospital for a cholecystectomy. The surgery has been explained by the ward doctor. The nursing assessment should include the pain history:

N. Have your gallstones given you any discomfort in the past?

P. Yes, I had an attack of pain about three months ago.

N. How would you describe the pain at that time?

P. It was very severe, like a colic; it made me feel sick as well.

N. Can you show me where you felt this pain?

P. It was right round my chest, but worse here, in front, just under my breast bone.

N. Do you remember when the pain began?

P. It came on after my tea, just when I sat down to watch the telly. It started suddenly and lasted for nearly two hours.

N. Was the pain the same all the time, or did it vary?

P. Well, it came and went a bit, but most of the time it was pretty bad – I've never known anything to match it anyway.

N. How did you feel when the pain began?

P. At first I was frightened, it fair took my breath away, and I thought perhaps I was having a heart attack, then I sort of got used to it. The wife got some of her Milk of Magnesia tablets. They eased it a bit.

N. Was there anything else that helped?

P. Yes, being sick. After that, the pain went altogether, then I just felt exhausted.

N. What do you think your wife felt about all this?

P. She said it was probably indigestion – that's why she gave me some tablets. But I think it put the wind up her a bit, so I decided to see the doctor next morning.

N. Have you had a similar pain since the attack you have told me about?

P. Well, not nearly so severe, but I've had heartburn and indigestion and find that I can't eat fried foods like before. Still, I've lost some weight with not eating fatty stuff – so there's some good come of it!

N. How do you feel about having to have an operation for your gallstones.

P. Well it's obvious that it's got to be done – I'd do anything rather than have a pain like that again. My neighbour had the same trouble, had the operation and got on famously; says he has never felt better, so I'm not too worried.

N. That's good, I'm sure you will get on well too, Mr Brown. Tell me, do you have any other aches, pains or discomforts which cause you any difficulty?

P. No, apart from the gallstones I'm as fit as a fiddle!

A conversation along these lines enables the nurse to gain a reasonable assessment of how the pain was, and is at present, when it occurs, where the pain is and the effect it has on the patient. It should be possible to ascertain the reaction to the pain and the patient's general attitude to the impending operation.

Notes following this conversation might read:

Pain assessment: Patient first experienced sudden onset of severe epigastric pain three months ago. Expressed fear as to cause before diagnosis was made. Pain relieved by vomiting and antacids. At present suffers from indigestion and heartburn, relieved by antacids. Has positive attitude to surgery but no previous experience of hospital or operations.

Plan: Discuss preparations for surgery and likely postoperative effects to avoid anxiety about the unknown and unexpected. Assure patient that analgesics will be readily available for wound discomfort – encourage Mr Brown to report any pain postoperatively.

Give low fat diet before surgery.

May require antacids for indigestion.

Sometimes the assessment of pain is not so straightforward and the nurse has to use ingenuity to encourage the patient to give the information:

Mrs Hide, a 48-year-old widow, had been admitted to the surgical ward from the out-patient department. Two years previously she had undergone surgery, having an anterior resection of the colon for carcinoma. It is clearly stated in her notes that she was told at the time of her discharge from hospital that 'she had a tumour which has been removed'. Her only close relation is a married daughter living in the Far East. The referral had been made by the GP and, according to his letter, Mrs Hide had visited him because of abdominal pain and weight loss.

The nursing assessment of pain proved more difficult in this case:

N. I'd like to ask you about your pain now, Mrs Hide.

P. Where? In my back?

N. Does your back hurt? – Can you show me where?

P. Well, I've had trouble on and off for years, but you learn to live with these things, don't you? My mother used to say, it's no good interfering with nature.

N. What do you find helps your back?

P. I used to go swimming but I haven't felt much like it recently.

N. Is your back a problem for you all the time?

P. No, only occasionally. I sometimes wake up feeling stiff but it usually wears off during the morning. I don't take any tablets or anything. It's really not much of a problem.

N. Have you any pain anywhere else?

P. It's just that I feel so weak – you know I've lost a lot of weight.

N. How has your tummy been feeling since the last operation?

P. Well it feels pretty rough just now, to be honest.

N. Do you mean that it hurts?

P. I get these cramps – feels like someone is squeezing my gut.

N. Can you tell me how bad this squeezing is?

P. Oh, I should say it's *very* bad and sometimes it goes on for hours. You know after I had that *abscess* done it was sore for a while . . .

N. But this is a different kind of discomfort isn't it, Mrs Hide?

P. Yes dear – it made me feel faint at times.

N. Do these cramps happen at any particular time?

P. No, and the thing is, I don't know what to do when they come. I held a hot water bottle once or twice, and I tried going to the toilet – do you think I've got another abscess? They said last time it was nothing to worry about. I do want to be well, my daughter and the grandchildren are coming at Easter – she's married to an oil man, they are very rich.

N. You must be looking forward to seeing them all. I think the Doctor asked you to come into hospital today so that we can see why you are getting these cramps. We want to help the pain so I'd like to ask you a bit more about it, then we can work out the best ways of making you more comfortable while you have the investigations.

P. That would be a relief, once or twice I thought I would go crazy. In the last couple of days the cramps have never left me properly. I tried to ignore it but it beat me in the end so I went to the doctor.

In this case history the patient was very reluctant to admit to her pain, in fact she never used the word 'pain' during the whole conversation. The nurse followed her lead in steering the conversation, which included a red herring from the patient, who tried to interest the nurse in her back, at the start of the interview. Although Mrs Hide had been told that her previous surgery was for a tumour, she referred to it as an abscess, presumably denying to herself the possibility of a recurrence. Her denial and unwillingness to talk about the pain associated with her abdomen was almost certainly for the same reason. Before investigation it would be impossible to be sure about the cause of the current problems and in such a case the nurse has to avoid using words which might be interpreted, or misinterpreted, by the patient, who subconsciously needs an answer. Having taken the time to establish a rapport and feeling of trust, the nurse can then proceed with a full assessment, to answer the essential questions – how, when, where, and the effects of the pain, so that she will then be able to plan appropriate care.

OBSERVING THE EFFECTS OF ACUTE PAIN

Surgical nurses are frequently able to observe patients' reactions to pain directly. Acute pain is usually associated with some physiological and behavioural changes.

Pain of *moderate to severe intensity* may be accompanied by the following physiological signs:

Pallor
Sweating
Increased heart rate
Increased respiratory rate and shallow breathing
Muscular tension/restlessness
Elevated blood pressure.

Pain which is *very* intense is frequently accompanied by:
Pallor
Decreased blood pressure
Decreased heart rate
Nausea and vomiting
Weakness and fainting
Possible loss of consciousness.

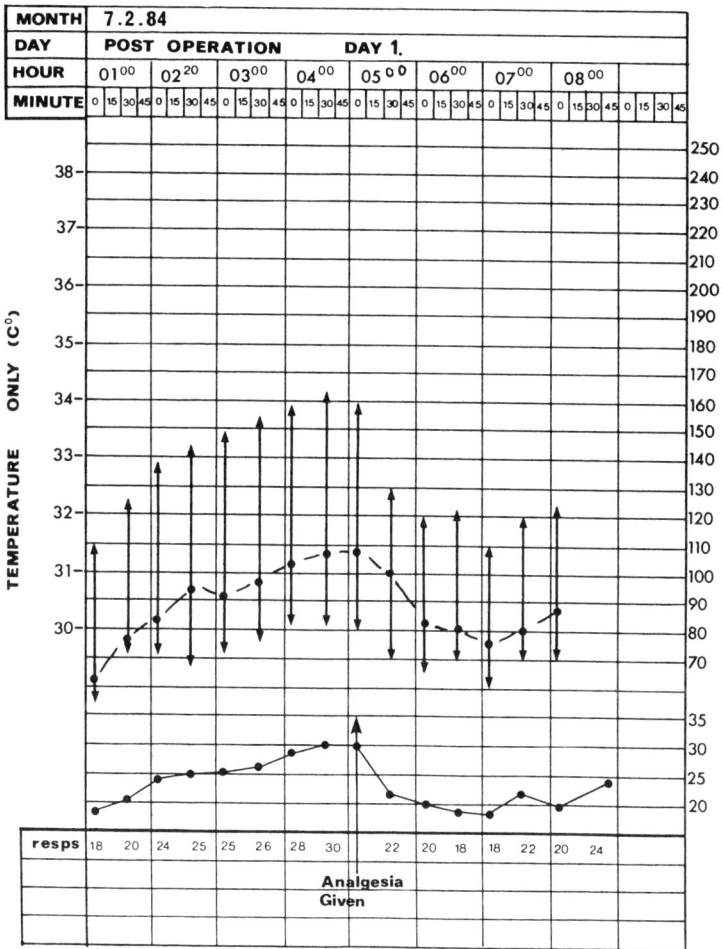

Fig. 4/3   Observation of the physiological signs of pain. This patient had been receiving continuous analgesia via an intravenous pump. During the night the equipment failed. As the effect of the analgesic wore off the postoperative pain level intensified and caused a steady increase in pulse rate, blood pressure and respiration rate. When analgesia was given at 0500 the beneficial effects were seen within half an hour of administration

The behavioural changes which may accompany pain include the following:

Adopting a posture to minimise the pain (drawing up of knees or lying rigidly)

Moaning or making other sounds to indicate discomfort

Crying or appearing frightened

Lying quietly, afraid of being touched

Grimacing and clenching jaws and/or fists, worried expression, closing eyes, pursed lips

Perspiring

Holding the painful area with hands.

Observation of the physiological and behavioural signs together with sympathetic questioning of patients in pain will enable the nurse to gain greater understanding of the individual's problem (Fig. 4/3). Patients with postoperative pain exhibit varying behaviours. The nurse must remember that every patient is an individual with a variety of physical, emotional and intellectual needs and life-experiences, all of which affect his current pain.

An assessment of postoperative pain is necessary to establish the best way of helping the patient. Sympathetic enquiry and questioning should be used to establish the severity of the pain being experienced and the degree of effectiveness of specific remedies previously offered. When assessing the effectiveness of drugs, it is important for the nurse to ask about any undesirable side-effects as well as the analgesic efficacy.

Case history

A patient who had minor surgery for a breast abscess was prescribed and given an injection of morphine two hours postoperatively for wound discomfort. The morphine provided complete pain relief but the patient experienced severe nausea and vomiting following the injection. This side-effect was much more upsetting for the patient than the wound pain. After consultation with the medical staff the analgesic prescription was changed, and no further morphine was given. The nausea settled and the wound discomfort was well controlled with an oral analgesic of moderate strength, no untoward side-effects occurred after the change in prescription.

The variability of patients' responses to pain is discussed in Chapter 5.

BIBLIOGRAPHY

Merskey, H. et al (1979). Pain terms: a list with definitions and notes on usage. *Pain*, **79,** 6, 249.

Jacox, A. (1979). Assessing pain. *American Journal of Nursing*, **79,** 5, 895.

Wolfer, J. and Davis, C. (1970). Assessment of surgical patients' pre-operative emotional condition and postoperative welfare. *Nursing Research*, **195**, 402.

Chapter Five

PREPARATION FOR SURGERY

People admitted to hospital for surgery are likely to be apprehensive, anxious or frightened. The amount of anxiety experienced pre-operatively is not necessarily influenced by the nature or extent of the anticipated surgery. For those without previous experience of a stay in hospital, a surgical ward with its strange and sometimes frightening equipment, and the sight of very ill patients with whom they may have to share a temporary bedroom, are likely to increase apprehension. Patients without previous experience of hospital cannot know what to expect, few seem to ask about what will happen to them, perhaps because they are not given sufficient opportunity or encouragement.

Facing the prospect of an operation places the patient in a situation which has a considerable element of the unknown. Having submitted to the advice of the surgeon and entered hospital it may seem to him that he has arrived on to a conveyor belt with little or no opportunity for open, relaxed discussion about the forthcoming events. The anxieties felt by many, though often not appreciated or expressed, include the fear of pain, having an anaesthetic, and worry about the outcome of the operation. Preparation for this event requires skill and understanding.

First impressions may be very important for those entering hospital for an operation. Frequently, patients are delayed by the admitting procedures, so by the time they reach the ward they may already be frustrated and anxious. When one has a visitor to one's home one extends a welcome and offers hospitality. When a patient arrives on a hospital ward the nurse can extend the same courtesy to make him feel welcome. This means that the patient is shown not only his bed and locker but is also introduced to other patients close by. He may be shown where the facilities of the ward are and told about the general routine: when and where meals will be served and how to get help. Whenever possible, new patients should be given a bed in a suitable environment: to offer a fit patient space next to an extremely ill one would be likely to induce stress in the new patient. Sometimes, this is unavoidable, and in such circumstances the nurse must offer explanation and reassurance.

The experiences of those who have had previous surgery will determine attitudes to the proposed operation. Some patients may bring memories with them which are unpleasant. For those people who have not previously required surgery there may be fear, as many are regaled with tales of alarm from well-meaning friends and relations. Before, during, and after the operation, there will be a multidisciplinary team involved with the total care of individual patients. Clearly the nurse occupies a position of considerable responsibility in identifying and meeting the needs of patients at all these times.

THE NURSE'S ROLE

Assessment

In recent years the Nursing Process has been widely introduced. This approach to nursing allows patients to receive care which is planned and evaluated to meet their individual needs and problems.

The first stage of the process is a nursing assessment during which the nurse can convey to the patient her interest in him as a person. Data are collected and then used to plan appropriate care. For patients who are being assessed prior to surgery the present pain history should be discussed together with the patients' reactions to painful situations (see Chapter 4).

Surgical wards are busy places and detailed assessment takes time, but the time spent pre-operatively is often well rewarded, with both the patient and the nurse benefiting from planned care. Most patients are part of a family so whenever possible try to include a close relative or friend who has accompanied the patient to hospital, for they too need reassurance that the surgery will not cause undue suffering. Figure 5/1 a-d is an example of nursing process assessment sheets.

When an opportunity is given to talk to the nurse, a great deal of relevant information can be obtained by both patient and nurse (Fig. 5/2). Anxieties which might otherwise not be recognised can be discussed.

GENERAL HEALTH HISTORY and PREVIOUS HOSPITAL ADMISSIONS
(note allergies chronic illnesses, etc.)

Vagotomy + Gastroenterostomy 1959
Laminectomy - 2 years ago.
Chronic back pain since last operation
No other chronic problems.

PRESENT HISTORY and REASON FOR ADMISSION

Sharp + stabbing abdominal pain for past 2/52 relieved by
vomiting. Investigated by physicians: gastroscopy revealed
Pyloric Stenosis
Some abdominal discomfort for past 2/12. Has been taking
DF118 × 8 tabs daily for back pain.

Antrectomy scheduled for 11.4.83.

GENERAL PHYSICAL ASSESSMENT ON ADMISSION: (Brief details of physical state including mobility, conscious
level, respiration, state of skin and mouth, disabilities, communication problems, prostheses and other significant
nursing problems).

Decreased mobility due to severe muscle wasting, back
and left leg. Unable to walk without crutches following
laminectomy.
  Looks pale
Eyesight + hearing - no problems
Own teeth - well cared for
Skin looks healthy
Communicates well.

Temperature: 36.5°C Pulse: 72   Respirations: 20   B/P: 130/70 Weight: 68 Kg

Urinalysis: Height (if applicable):   Norton Scale:
        NAD

GENERAL PSYCHOLOGICAL ASSESSMENT ON ADMISSION:
(Brief details of emotional state including any worries).

Appears anxious - states that his biggest problem is
depression - has a feeling that he will never be really well
again. Is worried about the outcome of proposed surgery
having had previous experience of 'failed' laminectomy
Has been feeling 'low' for months - has not received
medication or treatment for depression

Fig. 5/1 a.b.c.d.   Nursing assessment sheets

COMPLETE THE FOLLOWING ONLY IF APPROPRIATE

PAIN:
    ① Lower back and left leg
    Where ② Abdomen
    Type ① Dull ache (constant) ② Acute, severe stabbing (intermittent)
    Relieved by: ① DF118 ② vomiting

SLEEP:
    Normal Pattern: 2-3 hrs /night usually sitting in a chair
    Helped by: changed position. No sedation taken.

NUTRITION (Diet/Fluids):
    Normal/special diet: Ate normal diet until recently. Since vomiting +
    Preferences: pain had enjoyed a raw egg in milk.

ELIMINATION:
    Bladder problems: None

    Bowel problems: None. B.o. daily

    Laxative used at home: None

OTHER RELEVANT INFORMATION, e.g. Activity and movement, past work life, recreation activities.

Worked as a caretaker for old peoples home. Sustained back injury whilst working in 1981 and has not been able to work since slipped disc. Gastric problems were thought to be due partly to high analgesic intake.

Lives with wife and 3 of his six children. Wife has a heart condition and 'bad nerves' Three children away from home - working and married. Came into hospital on his own.

Activity very limited - breeds cage birds and watches T.V, not interested in reading.

Most comfortable when sitting in a high backed chair Coping financially with some help from the grown up children.

SURNAME   FIRST NAME   REGIS. NO.

WHAT PATIENT and/or FAMILY UNDERSTAND ABOUT HIS/HER CONDITION

Realises the need to get gastric problem sorted out - requests more information about exactly what will be done at

REACTION OF PATIENT and/or FAMILY TO HOSPITAL ADMISSION.   Operation

Patient regards treatment as necessary, but is 'scared' and depressed.

HOW LONG DOES PATIENT EXPECT TO BE IN HOSPITAL

10 days

WHERE WILL THE PATIENT GO ON DISCHARGE:

Home

HOW DOES THE PATIENT EXPECT TO GET HOME:

Son will fetch by car.

HOME ENVIRONMENT: (Factors affecting future welfare of the patient, e.g. stairs, location of toilet, social services and community services received)

Lives in a council house, bathroom upstairs, but ground floor toilet.
Unable to bath without help - recent application for a grant for downstairs bathroom failed.
Handrails fixed to stairs and back door. Level garden.

No social services - wife at home + not working

Social worker visits family, involved since last surgery.

INFORMATION OBTAINED FROM: Patient

SIGNATURE: DATE: 9.4.83

SURNAME		FIRST NAME	REGIS NO:	
DATE and PROBLEM NUMBER	NURSING PROBLEM or POTENTIAL PROBLEM	NURSING CARE PLAN		REVIEW DATE and INITIALS
9.4.83.		Ask medical staff to give more information		
1.	Anxiety about Surgery	Explain procedures and preparations.		
2.	Pain	Assess and evaluate current pain and pain relief - ask patient to use chart. Involve patient in his treatment & establish aggravating factors.		
3.	Poor Sleep pattern	Involve physiotherapist - will require suitable chair beside bed. Offer night sedation.		
4.	Vomiting / possible Weight loss	Monitor diet & fluid intake / output. Record weight daily. Offer nourishing fluids. Give anti emetic if prescribed.		10. 4. 84
5.	Decrease in mobility due to hospitalisation	Encourage activity pre-operatively		
6.	General condition	Observe Temp & Pulse		
7.	Hygiene	Assist patient to bath.		
10.4.84.	PREPARATION FOR SURGERY			
1.	Increased anxiety - fear of surgery + anaesthesia	Give reassurance & full explanation of pre-op measures. Give pre-med as Kardex.		
2.	Anxiety about post op pain.	Discuss post-op analgesia with patient - encourage reporting of discomfort. Liaise with physio & reinforce breathing exercises.		
3.	Rest	Encourage night sedation pre operatively.		
4.	Adequate Hydration	I.V. fluids commenced, running as Kardex - keep accurate record of intake / output.		
5.	Mobility	Practise movement for post op period with physio.		
6. } 7 }	Preparation of bowel and skin	Give 2 suppositories Nocte. Abdominal & chest shave. Give bath after shave.		
8.	Concern of relatives	Inform of time of surgery & when to enquire - reassure and give explanations about post-op care.		

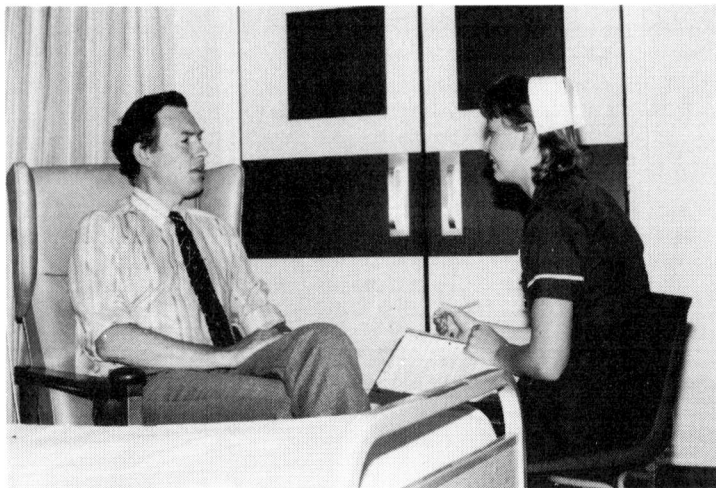

Fig. 5/2   Nursing assessment with a pre-operative patient

Case history
A middle-aged man was admitted to a surgical ward for the second stage of a lower abdominal operation, the first operation having been performed three months earlier. During the discussion pre-operatively he confided that he felt he had 'suffered to an inhuman degree in the hands of the physiotherapist'. After the first operation he developed a severe chest infection which had required very active physiotherapy. Before the second operation the ward physiotherapist visited this intelligent and sensible man and together they discussed the need for deep breathing and established a relationship of trust. With the knowledge that those caring for him were anticipating that he might have chest complications again and were taking active preventive steps, the anticipated pain was put into perspective. He was assured that pain-killing drugs would be readily available. Had the facts of his previous experiences not been acquired the actions taken may not have been thought necessary, especially as this patient appeared quite willing to submit himself to further surgery.

Those who have had a previous painful experience should be given the opportunity to vent their feelings. Assurance must be given that relief of pain will not be neglected, and these patients should be encouraged to report any pain after surgery.

Explanation

An account of how the operation day will be managed may help to relieve the fear of the unknown. The reasons for various preparations should be given and, in particular, nursing practices such as moving beds from one part of the ward to another should be outlined.

Nurses cannot always answer specific medical questions but should enable information to be obtained by involving other members of the team. When a promise is made to obtain information by asking the doctor, it is the nurse's duty to ensure that he responds. The patient's query must be passed on to the medical staff and with it a request for the doctor to see the patient himself. If the doctor is unable to do this immediately then the nurse should relay an appropriate message to the patient, informing him of the time when the doctor will be available.

Explanations about pre-operative procedures are essential. When the patient knows why something uncomfortable needs to be done, it is easier to accept. An enema could never be described as a pleasant procedure but it is often necessary, and if the recipient understands that this preparation will prevent complications later, he will be reassured.

Information

Should nurses withold information about the postoperative use of nasogastric tubes, infusions and drains because the prospect of them may increase anxiety? Hayward (1975) found that for the majority of patients, information provided a 'prescription against pain'. Lack of information may lead to increased anxiety which can cause more pain and suffering than perhaps need be the case.

What is actually said about the pain that is likely to occur following the operation will depend to some extent on the nurse's assessment of each individual patient. Some are eager for facts and precise details, perhaps wanting to know the name of the drug that might be used to help the pain, but others are content with the minimum of explanation.

All patients awaiting surgery may be told by nurses that they should not expect to have unnecessary pain. Some believe that discomfort and suffering are a necessary part of the healing process. The reverse is probably true, as pain may delay the return to normal of endocrine and metabolic changes which occur during and after surgery. This can delay healing and decrease resistance to infection as well as cause suffering; postoperative pain can have a profound effect on respiratory function, particularly after abdominal and thoracic surgery (see p. 71).

The effects of the anaesthetic and surgery upon the patient are numerous and will be different for every individual. It is not possible to tell patients specifically how they are likely to feel, but it is reasonable and sensible to explain in simple language some of the effects likely to be experienced.

Wound pain can be referred to as discomfort, or an ache. It should be stressed that any discomfort can be lessened by analgesics given before the pain becomes distressing, thus emphasising the need for the patient to report feelings and not hide discomfort. It is necessary to disturb postoperative patients to change their position in bed and to monitor vital signs. This should be explained, emphasising that between observations and turning, relaxation and sleep will be possible.

The nurse can tell pre-operative patients that some people experience a feeling of sickness after surgery. The nausea is usually short-lived and may be helped by deep breathing. Encourage the patient to call for the nurse should he experience this problem and explain that medication will be available if the nausea persists.

When it is expected that drainage tubes will be used, the nurse can explain their function and at the same time warn of the type of drainage, to prevent the patient from panicking after surgery.

As it is now common practice to be nursed in a recovery ward for the immediate postoperative period, patients appreciate being told about this. To wake up in an unexpected environment may induce panic. Quite reasonably the patient may ask 'Why am I here?' and may, logically enough, assume that something must have gone wrong. Even if the recovery room is not remembered, the shock at realising the length of time away from the ward might lead to a similar worried reaction.

Oxygen is frequently given in the recovery period after any operation. When it is anticipated that oxygen will be given postoperatively, the patient should be told beforehand that this is a routine procedure, as some people associate oxygen masks with very serious illness or even death. Explanation by the nurse that the oxygen will assist and aid recovery after a general anaesthetic, ensures that the patient does not worry about what might have gone wrong during the operation.

Most patients awaiting surgery are encouraged to be up and around the ward looking after their own needs. After the operation most will be dependent on the nursing staff for hours or even days. The ward nurses must make sure that patients are familiar with the nurse-call system before the operation, and on return to the ward following surgery, that they are able to reach the call-button.

Intensive care
In many hospitals patients who have undergone major surgical procedures are nursed in special intensive care units.

When this is anticipated, it is helpful for the patient to meet and talk with a nurse from that unit. If possible the patient should be enabled to visit the unit, when discussion about the equipment used and specialised care can take place. This assists in the emotional and practical preparation of the patient. During recovery, the familiar faces of the nurses and an understanding of the procedures used are likely to be helpful and comforting.

GROUPS AT RISK FROM INADEQUATE PREPARATION

Patients with existing problems
It is not unusual for people who have chronic health problems to require surgery. Those who live with a disabling condition often cope remarkably when at home by adapting their lives to diminish the effects of their handicap. When the need for surgery forces such a person into a hospital ward, much of that support may be missing. Many disabling conditions are painful and this group of patients often depends on regular doses of analgesic and anti-inflammatory drugs to control the effects of conditions affecting the joints, tendons, cartilage and muscles. The non-steroidal anti-inflammatory drugs (NSAID) reduce inflammation and therefore pain (see Chapter 8). They are widely used for rheumatism and arthritis.

If it is anticipated that anticoagulants may be used during or after surgery, then any patient taking one of the NSAID group will have to stop before the surgery. The reason for this is that the anticoagulant is potentiated by the non-steroidal anti-inflammatory drugs. This is because the NSAIDs have the ability to displace warfarin and similar drugs from proteins to which they bind in the blood. Once displaced, they become proportionately more active, leading to bleeding and may be especially dangerous if the NSAIDs' other side-effects such as peptic ulceration or gastro-intestinal bleeding also occur.

When the analgesic anti-inflammatory drugs are stopped because of impending surgery, patients may miss their effects and are likely to stiffen up. In addition, the period of relative immobility following the surgical procedure is likely to aggravate this problem. The management of pain following surgery for these people may be difficult.

Pain relief for both the operative wound and the underlying chronic condition has to be provided by drugs which do not interfere with the clotting mechanism and do not induce a tendency to bleeding.

Nursing observation and accurate history taking are essential preoperatively to ensure the most effective means of help after the surgery.

The nurse should also enlist the help of other specialists preoperatively. Visits from a physiotherapist and occupational therapist can help the caring team to understand what goals to aim for in the recovery phase. Patients who have a chronic pain problem may not respond as readily to postoperative analgesics. For many, a degree of tolerance develops to the drugs which they require and for this group it may be necessary to allow for larger than usual doses of analgesic to be prescribed. This problem may be overcome by the use of a flexible prescription allowing for dosage adjustment according to the patient's needs (see Chapter 7).

Emergencies

Sometimes the need for immediate surgery means that a planned nursing approach is not possible. Trauma surgery often has to take place within minutes of arrival at the accident department.

Acute surgical emergencies frequently require almost immediate surgical intervention. Faced with this prospect, patients have little or no time to prepare. Anxiety is often experienced about work, family and financial affairs. Those requiring emergency surgery must be aware that the illness is already serious. Fear of the operation, and its outcome, together with the anxiety of being unexpectedly ill, are added to the acute pain which may already exist.

Nurses working in accident and emergency departments, transit wards and theatre reception areas should be familiar with procedures in other parts of their own hospitals. Explanations and information should be given whenever possible. This will decrease the anxiety and reassure both patients and their relations.

The time spent in hospital before an operation may be five minutes or five days. In either case the patient has a need for emotional support and explanations. Pre-operative patients are very dependent on nursing and medical staff and are usually aware that they will be even more dependent after the operation.

When care is planned with the individual, and explanations have been given about what will happen and why, the patient is likely to feel secure and will leave the ward on his way to theatre trusting in the nurses' ability to continue this care and support after the operation.

THE ROLE OF OTHERS

Physiotherapist

The ward nurse and physiotherapist can assist each other by working closely together for the benefit of patients. In her initial assessment of the pre-operative patient the nurse may identify the 'at risk' patient who would benefit from pre-operative instruction and therapy.

Pre-operative physiotherapy as a routine is not always possible, indeed research has shown that in the 'normal' patient it does not alter the occurrence of postoperative chest infections (Nichols and Howell, 1970). However, for patients who already have impaired respiratory function, pre-operative physiotherapy can be very helpful. Intensive treatment over a period of days, monitoring the effects of the treatment, ensures that surgery is performed when the patient has achieved the maximum possible function.

When a pre-operative visit is undertaken, the physiotherapist has an opportunity to make her own assessment of the patient and to get to know him. She is likely to stress the importance of deep breathing to minimise the risk of chest infections and can teach the most effective ways of achieving good respiratory function (Fig. 5/3).

The type of anticipated surgery will determine specific pre-operative instructions. Knowing how to breathe effectively is important for any patient having general surgery but for those undergoing major abdominal, upper abdominal and thoracic operations it requires greater emphasis. For patients awaiting orthopaedic surgery the physiotherapist may concentrate more on movement, mobility and relaxation in preparation for the recovery phase.

The nurse has an important role in reinforcing the physiotherapist's explanations and instruction; she can also encourage patients to practise their exercises in the pre-operative period. These instructions can include showing patients before operation how to support their wound when coughing (Fig. 5/4), practising the best way to move around in bed and practising foot and leg movements to maintain circulation.

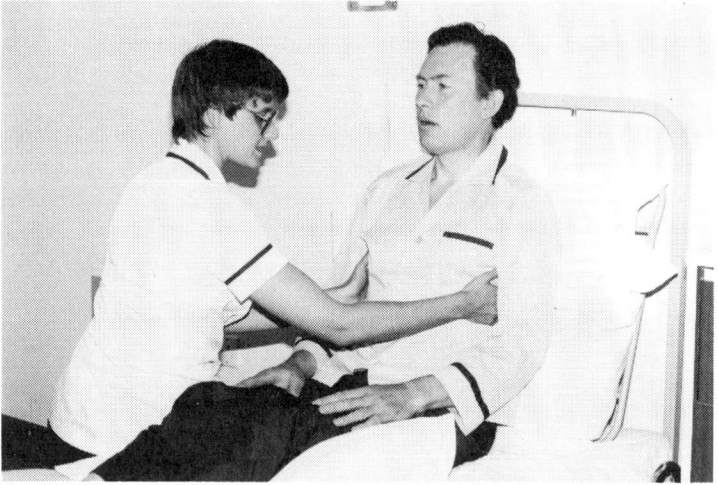

Fig. 5/3   Pre-operative breathing instruction from the physiotherapist

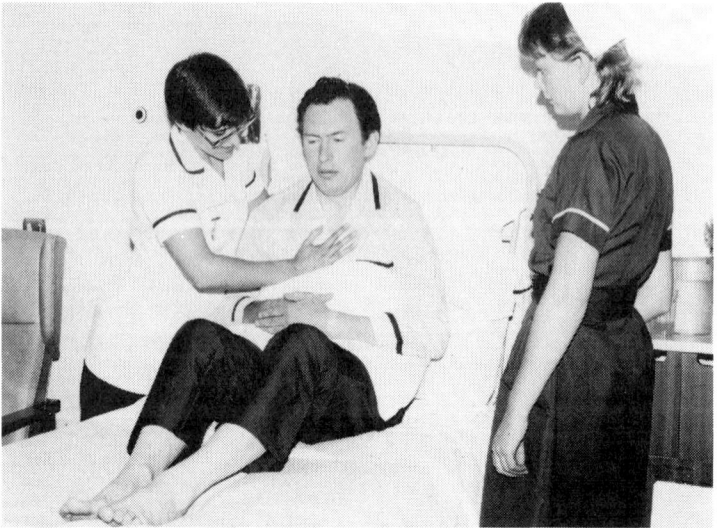

Fig. 5/4   Showing how to support an abdominal wound while coughing

Surgeon

Most patients arriving on a ward for a planned stay in hospital are aware of the reason for surgery. Having previously been seen in the out-patient department, most will have had an explanation from the surgeon they saw. However, it is not unusual for several members of the surgical team to interview, examine, and sometimes pronounce judgement on a patient's condition. This may lead to confusion and uncertainty.

The practice of giving each patient a written list of the names and designation of the doctors who will be involved with their care on the ward is appreciated. The house officer is usually the doctor responsible for ensuring that the patient understands the nature and purpose of the operation and who usually obtains the written consent for surgery.

Anaesthetist

A pre-operative visit by the anaesthetist should allay the anxiety which many people associate with being put to sleep and waking up again – the only parts of the operation of which most are aware. If this takes place the anaesthetist may tell the pre-operative patient about the availability of postoperative analgesics for he is usually responsible for prescribing such drugs and this aspect of care should be expanded and reinforced by the nurse. It is most important that the patient knows that analgesics will be available.

Pre-operative medication is often prescribed by the anaesthetist. The drugs used most commonly are the benzodiazepines and the opiates. The former group, which include diazepam and lorazepam are primarily anxiolytics and afford the patient relaxation and some sedation prior to surgery. The opiates give most patients a feeling of well-being and sedation when used pre-operatively. Sometimes a combination of drugs may be given, a sedative or hypnotic agent together with hyoscine (scopolamine) or atropine; the latter two drugs serve to reduce secretions and patients should be warned that they may experience a dry feeling in the mouth. The non-opiate sedatives are usually prescribed to be administered with a small amount of water and are given orally 1–2 hours before the patient leaves the ward. The opiates are more frequently given by intramuscular injection.

Some anaesthetists also prescribe an alkaline mixture to be taken orally prior to the induction of the anaesthetic. When given, this neutralises stomach acidity so that in the event of vomiting during induction, potentially dangerous acid secretions do not enter the lungs.

REFERENCES

Hayward, J. (1975). *Information – A Prescription Against Pain*. Study of Nursing Care, Series Two, Royal College of Nursing, London.

Nichols, P. J. R. and Howell, B. (1970). Routine pre- and postoperative physiotherapy. Results of a trial. *Rheumatology and Physical Medicine*, **10**, 321–36.

BIBLIOGRAPHY

Bruegel, M. (1971). Relationship of pre-operative anxiety to perception of postoperative pain. *Nursing Research*, **20**, 26.

Leigh, J. et al (1977). Effect of pre-operative anaesthetic visit on anxiety. *British Medical Journal*, **2**, 987.

Well, N. (1984). Responses to acute pain and the nursing implications. *Journal of Advanced Nursing*, **9**, 51–8.

Chapter Six

RESPIRATORY FUNCTION AND SURGERY

When a patient is anaesthetised a marked decrease in lung capacity is seen, though exactly why this should happen is not known. This effect lasts for a variable period after surgery. It tends to be of minor significance and of short duration following peripheral, and head and neck surgery, but may have profound effects following abdominal, upper abdominal and thoracic operations. The effect is most marked in the immediate postoperative period and may not return to normal for 7 to 10 days.

Pain increases the reduction of lung capacity and there appears to be a direct association between the severity of pain being experienced, the fall in lung capacity and the duration of this decrease.

Carbon dioxide (CO_2) production in the tissues is related to the basal metabolic rate and level of activity. Most postoperative patients have a normal metabolic rate and in this respect CO_2 production remains fairly constant. CO_2 excretion from the lungs is related to the minute volume of ventilation, which is the product of the rate and depth of respiration (tidal volume).

A postoperative patient with reduced tidal volume after major abdominal or thoracic surgery compensates by an increase in the rate of respiration. When the normal minute volume of ventilation is not maintained, the CO_2 level in the blood rises. This causes peripheral vasodilation; patients may look pink and healthy but the CO_2 retention causes confusion and sleepiness. CO_2 retention causes a respiratory acidosis which may cause cardiac arrhythmias.

The reduced functional residual capacity of the lungs, which is worse with increasing age, may also cause collapse of airways and alveoli. These collapsed airways, though not expanded and oxygenated, are still perfused with blood, with the result that venous blood enters the left ventricle of the heart without being oxygenated and so enters the arterial system, diluting the oxygenated blood with venous blood. This leads to arterial hypoxia, further acidosis, and a decrease in cerebral and other vital organ functions. Collapse of the airways also leads to the inability of lung secretions to move upward through the respiratory tract on the epithelium. The secretions stay 'dammed-up' and become stagnant, inviting infection. The bases of the lungs are the most commonly affected, giving rise to postoperative basal pneumonia.

When the tidal volume is increased, the airways are kept open. Deep breathing enables patients to cough effectively, which encourages secretions to move upward. Deep breathing also ventilates portions of the lung otherwise not receiving oxygen and so reduces hypoxia.

Limited movement and reluctance to breathe deeply because of pain also result in reduced respiratory function and predisposes to chest infections. Pain relief makes it easier for the patient to increase his lung capacity, with effective deep breathing and coughing. In turn, this gives improved CO_2 excretion and an increase in tidal volume. The result of this is to decrease the risk of chest infection and also to increase the performance of the vital organs of the body by enabling the arterial circulation to remain fully oxygenated. This in turn aids general recovery from surgery and promotes wound healing.

Chapter Seven

THE NURSE'S ROLE IN THE
MANAGEMENT OF ACUTE PAIN

Most people with a painful condition expect the operation to cure the pain. This is generally true, but the first and most obvious effect of surgery will be that the patient will probably have even more pain than before. For others, surgery will produce pain where there was none before.

INDICATIONS FOR PAIN RELIEF

If the patient is able to report that he has pain, then the nurse immediately knows that there is a need both to assess the pain and provide appropriate relief. It must be stressed that some patients are unable or unwilling to communicate their subjective feelings, in which case the nurse must use her skills to evaluate the objective signs indicating the need for analgesia.

Signs of acute pain

The intensity of postoperative pain is likely to vary with the extent and site of the surgery; upper abdominal, thoracic and major rectal operations tend to produce the most severe and distressing pain. Acute pain may be accompanied by physiological signs (see p. 52). Pallor and sweating are frequently seen, the facial expression is often tense. The patient with acute severe pain is often restless and may cry out, but following surgery the reaction to the pain is not always verbalised. He may lie tense and rigid effectively splinting the painful wound. Breathing often becomes shallow and increases in respiration rate and heart rate are usually seen. These signs may be accompanied by a rise in blood pressure. Acute pain almost always produces anxiety which in its turn heightens awareness of pain.

ATTITUDES TO PAIN RELIEF

Empathy is the power of projecting one's personality into the object of contemplation so that it can be fully understood. Most nurses are young and few have themselves suffered pain similar to that which may result from major surgery. This lack of common experience can make it difficult to comprehend fully the patient's experience of pain.

Sympathy can be defined as mental participation in another's trouble so that compassion and a favourable attitude of mind towards that person is achieved. A lack of empathy may cause an inappropriately low level of sympathy towards the patient in pain.

Perception of pain in others varies greatly in individuals, and the interpretation which a nurse places on the pain reported by her patient will affect the way in which she responds to it. A young man who has to have his leg amputated following an accident in which he was an innocent victim is likely to arouse a sympathetic response, whereas numerous reports of pain from a middle-aged man following a minor procedure may invoke less compassionate feelings.

The nurse as pain reliever

It is necessary for patients to know that the nurse cares. Too often in the surgical setting, relief of pain equates only with the administration of analgesics – for every nurse it should mean more. It is the nurse who, hour by hour, day by day, assists the patient in coping with pain and who attempts to provide relief whenever possible. In order to do this the nurse must first recognise that the patient is in pain and then evaluate the extent and cause of the suffering so that appropriate relief can be given.

Acute severe pain following surgery generally requires the use of moderate or strong analgesics. Such medication will be enhanced by the way in which the specific remedy is given by the nurse. An uncomfortable patient who requests pain relief while lying on a crumpled sheet may receive an injection, but if at the same time the discomfort from his position in bed is not relieved, then the nurse has failed in her role. If a patient asks for something for the pain and the nurse responds by going to ask and then does not return, either with the relief, or an explanation as to why nothing can be given, then the patient will feel that his pain is not important to the nurse. Patients in pain are perhaps more sensitive to the way others regard them. Being ill and in pain can produce a profound feeling of vulnerability.

When care is taken in such a way that the patient feels emotionally supported, confident and secure, then both patient and nurse will benefit: the nurse by deriving satisfaction, and the patient, because the nurse's attitude has generated a considerable amount of placebo analgesia (see p.146). When the patient knows that his reports of pain will be met with acceptance and belief, he is much less anxious. The suffering is lessened and usually the intensity of his pain also subsides as a result of such an interaction. A relationship of trust also enables the patient to communicate problems and report pain calmly.

Once the need for pain relief is established, delay in giving specific drugs should be avoided. If the pain is left unrelieved the accompanying anxiety is likely to increase the perception of pain and decrease tolerance to it. The analgesic will then be less effective. Most usually, analgesics are given by the intramuscular route in the immediate postoperative period. Drugs given in this way take from 10 to 20 minutes to start to work and, in the case of most, at least an hour to reach maximum effect. It is therefore necessary and important for the nurse to return to the patient to check the effects. This is reassuring for both and allows the nurse to evaluate the relief of pain. The analgesic effect of the prescribed medication may be monitored by using a pain relief chart (Fig. 7/1). Such charts provide a useful communication tool and can be made available for both doctors' and nurses' reference and discussion. When the medication is inadequate, the medical staff *must* be asked to review the prescription.

SAFETY OF PATIENTS

The administration of analgesia is the responsibility of the trained nurse and it is usually nurses who decide when to give analgesics. The desirable and undesirable effects of narcotics are discussed in Chapter 9. Nurses should have an understanding of these effects so that a rational decision is made in respect of the patient's safety. There are situations when the nurse may have to withold analgesia for a time, because to administer it could endanger the patient's life.

Respiratory depression

It is generally true that pain acts as a natural antagonist to the respiratory depression produced by narcotics. However, nurses caring for patients in acute pain must be aware that the patient may experience respiratory depression if he is either very susceptible to this effect (see Chapter 6), or if his pain suddenly subsides. Respiratory depression may also occur if the patient receives more than enough narcotic to relieve the pain, as doses in excess of what is needed for pain relief are capable of depressing respiration significantly.

Some sedation following the administration of narcotics is usual. Natural sleep also causes some degree of respiratory depression and the effects of sleep and the narcotic are additive. It is therefore vital that patients who are well sedated following the administration of narcotics are very carefully observed.

When a narcotic causes significant respiratory depression, the nurse may be able to get the patient to increase his rate and depth of breathing simply by instructing him to do so. The nurse should stay with the patient, call for assistance and ensure that the medical staff are informed. If the patient does not respond to instructions or is already in a coma then artificial respiration together with the administration of a narcotic antagonist, to reverse the depressant effect of the analgesic will be necessary.

Continued observation of the patient is essential following treatment for narcotic-induced respiratory depression. The effect of naloxone is relatively short compared to the depressant effect of the narcotic which can last for several hours, causing the patient to slip back again into respiratory depression and coma (see Chapter 9).

The most dangerous aspect of narcotic-induced respiratory depression is that the patient may go unobserved and therefore untreated. The nurse's role in preventing a disaster is one of watching carefully and instituting the appropriate treatment when necessary.

If pain is reported or the nurse, by her observations, feels that pain relief is indicated, she must reassure herself that it is safe to give the prescribed pain-relieving drug.

Low blood pressure
Patients recovering from anaesthesia after major surgery may already have a reduced blood pressure, due to blood loss or shock. The decision about whether or not to administer a narcotic on such occasions is a difficult one.

Fig. 7/1 (opposite)   A pain record. It can be filled in by the patient, or a nurse with the patient, and records the degree of pain being experienced and the relief afforded by an analgesic

PAIN RECORD

NAME	John Brown	HOSPITAL NUMBER	AB 1234	DATE 1. 2. 85

TIME	01^{00}	02^{00}	03^{00}	04^{00}	05^{00}	06^{00}	07^{00}	08^{00}	09^{00}	10^{00}	11^{00}	12^{00}	13^{00}	14^{00}	15^{00}	16^{00}	17^{00}	18^{00}	19^{00}	20^{00}	21^{00}	22^{00}	23^{00}	24^{00}
ANALGESIC i.m. morphine Name & Route	Dose 10 mg	Dose	Dose	Dose	Dose 15 mg	Dose	Dose	Dose	Dose 15 mg	Dose	Dose	Dose	Dose 15 mg	Dose	Dose	Dose	Dose 10 mg	Dose	Dose	Dose	Dose 10 mg	Dose	Dose	Dose

SEVERITY OF PAIN
- SEVERE
- MODERATE
- SLIGHT
- NONE or ASLEEP

AMOUNT OF PAIN RELIEF
- COMPLETE
- ALMOST COMPLETE
- MODERATE
- SLIGHT
- NONE

When circumstances permit, the best method of coping with the situation is to administer small amounts of narcotics intravenously, watching the effects carefully. Increase in circulating blood volume may be achieved by additional IV fluids given at the same time.

Continuous infusion

When analgesia is administered continuously using an infusion pump, careful monitoring of the infusion rate and of the effects of it on the respiration rate are essential. This can be conveniently recorded using a 'pump chart' (Fig. 7/2) which enables all the staff to see at a glance the drug being used, its route of administration and the total amount of the drug that the patient has received. In the event of respirations becoming significantly decreased, the nurses are instructed to switch off the analgesic infusion and inform the medical staff (see Chapter 13).

THE VARIABILITY OF PATIENTS' RESPONSES TO PAIN

Effective management of pain on a surgical ward requires that staff are aware of the variability of patients' responses to painful conditions.

Occasionally after major surgery, but more frequently following minor operations, patients genuinely have no pain and require no analgesia. The average patient will have a predictable amount of pain postoperatively which will last for a fairly predictable time after a specified operation.

The undemanding patient

Sometimes patients make fewer demands than expected. Nurses may marvel at a person's ability to be uncomplaining and think of such a patient as being very 'good'. The 'good' patient may be hiding or under-reporting pain, not wishing to make a fuss. In such a person, observation of the physiological signs indicating that pain is present, and careful enquiry are even more important. An increase in requests for pain relief is often seen during visiting times when patients may admit to those who know them best that they are suffering.

Some may be reluctant to ask for pain relief fearing that a request may bring recriminations from nursing staff. A situation can arise where the patient is afraid of the nurses and their reactions.

Comments like 'Your friend in the next bed had the same operation as you and he hasn't needed any pain-killers today' do nothing to help patients who may be in need of specific analgesia and other

NAME **N. Jones**   DATE **3.5.84**

NO. **B. 1212**

DRUG **Morphine 1mg/ml**   START TIME **11.00**

RATE OF INFUSION **3ml/hour**

ROUTE OF INFUSION **i.v.**

	ANALGESIA PUMP CHART			
TIME	Amount Remaining Syringe/Pump	Amount Infused in Past Hour	Total Infused	Respiration Rate
11.00	45ml	—	—	24
12.00	42ml	3ml	3ml	22
13.00	39ml	3ml	6ml	23
14.00	36ml	3ml	9ml	18
15.00	34ml	2ml	11ml	20
16.00	31ml	3ml	14ml	18
17.00	28ml	3ml	17ml	17
18.00	28ml	—	17	20
18.05	28ml ↑ Pump switched off by cleaner ↑			20
19.00	25ml	3ml	20ml	22
20.00	22ml	3ml	23ml	18

N.B. If Respiratory Rate falls below 12/min SWITCH OFF PUMP and inform Medical Staff.

Fig. 7/2   A pump chart for use with patients who are receiving continuous effusions of narcotics

comfort measures. Following surgery, most patients are psychologically dependent on those caring for them and they need the nurse to care.

A sad reflection on this was left by a middle-aged man following a haemorrhoidectomy when he wrote:

> Basically I was made to feel it was wrong to ask for pain-killers and was never offered. I asked twice, at times when I knew my bowels were about to open. It became a question of 'are you more afraid of the Sisters or of the pain.' Going to the toilet got steadily more painful not less.

The demanding patient

When a patient reports pain, perhaps in the absence of physiological signs, it may seem to the nurse that unreasonable demands are being made. Postoperative pain should *always* be regarded as genuine. It is essential to seek as much information as possible about the pain, so that appropriate relief may be given. Correct doses of analgesics can then be given at the right times and unnecessary pain-killers will not be required. Time spent seeking the reason for unusual demands for pain-relief is frequently rewarded.

Case history

John, a 28-year-old, previously fit, man was admitted to the ward at 0330 following an emergency appendicectomy. While in the operating theatre his wife had visited the ward leaving his suitcase with things he would need. At 0900 the same day he was sitting beside his bed looking distressed and uncomfortable. Two postoperative doses of narcotic analgesic had been given, one in the recovery room immediately after the operation, the second at 0800 hours. He was wearing only crumpled hospital trousers, and no jacket. The nurse looking after him reported that he was a 'demanding patient with a low pain threshold'. When asked about his pain John said 'It's awful, everything is awful – I can't see because I haven't got my glasses; I can't phone my wife to find out what has happened to my suitcase because I haven't any money – that's in the bag, and I'm having to sit here half-dressed.' It seemed likely that the cause of John's 'unreasonable demands' was the anxiety associated with his situation. John readily supplied the telephone number for his wife at her work and the lost suitcase was discovered. When he could see properly and dress appropriately John felt better, coped well, and made excellent progress, requiring only mild analgesia for his wound pain. If his nurse had taken a little more time to question her 'demanding patient' she would have allayed his distress, lowered his perception of pain and increased the effectiveness of the analgesic.

'Low pain-threshold' – the need to question why

The term pain-threshold is mistakenly used to describe pain-tolerance by many nurses. As mentioned in Chapter 1, the pain-threshold is the intensity of stimulation at which it becomes painful.

When postoperative patients demonstrate by their actions or demands that pain-relief is required, they are expressing their individual responses to the pain being experienced. Tolerance of pain differs greatly from one to another and may be affected by influences which can serve to heighten or decrease what is felt and reported.

There are two groups of patients whose responses to postoperative pain cause the most concern. The first of these groups may moan, scream and thrash about in bed in a great display of suffering. These patients are often labelled as having a 'low pain-threshold' with the result that staff may adopt a 'high threshold' of treatment for them. This common situation may be the result of the sociological background of the staff themselves, who might view any open and apparently uninhibited display of pain as a sign of weakness of character. Such a patient has a 'catch 22' problem as the staff underestimate his pain *because* of the display of suffering. The only way the patient could get treatment of his pain would be by reporting the pain less. These patients are difficult to treat because the usual subjective descriptions tend not to work. It is therefore more prudent to gauge the amount of pain with objective indicators, such as the ability to move freely, the ability to cough properly and to breathe deeply, if these would normally be affected by the wound pain. After some sort of objective assessment of the patient's pain has been made and steps taken to treat it, his suffering should also be relieved with both physical and psychological comforting.

The second difficult group concerns those patients in whom analgesics do not seem to be as effective as usual. In this case there are some general prescribing rules which may be helpful.

1. If a dose of analgesic does not work at all, either give more each time, or use a drug from a stronger group
2. If the analgesic works, but does not last long enough, either shorten the interval between each dose, or give a longer-acting analgesic of similar strength.

Poor pain tolerance

Sometimes patients continue to report pain despite general and specific nursing measures to alleviate it. The reasons for their continuing discomfort need assessment – the following groups are worthy of special consideration.

The elderly and the young: Age appears to affect the perception of pain. A 76-year-old farmer well known to one of the authors (JH), recently experienced an accident while getting down from a tractor, which caused him to rupture his testis. When this story was related to me I remarked that it must have been a very painful injury. He replied, 'Not nearly as painful as when I was kicked in the same place by a bull 50 years ago'. No doubt at the age of 26 the perception of pain was influenced not only by the possible effect that such an accident might have on his manhood, but also by the possibility of having to take time off work. At the age of 76 with all of life's experiences behind him, the tractor accident did not assume as much significance and the pain from it was put into a different perspective and perhaps became easier to tolerate. Because older people tend to report pain less they may receive fewer pain-killers, but this does not mean that they have less pain, merely that they do not display the same reactions to it.

It may not be surprising that younger people sometimes find pain hard to accept and tolerate, as their previous experiences of life may not have prepared them for it. The experience of severe pain may be bewildering and frightening, even unacceptable to some, who may also display resentment towards members of staff as being associated with the causes of the pain.

Cancer patients: The patient with cancer pain may have special problems as some will have had the unfortunate experience of not being believed about their pain prior to diagnosis. When surgery is performed for the treatment of cancer, patients are extremely anxious about the outcome of the operation. This anxiety may be reflected in demands for pain-relief.

When surgery confirms the presence of malignancy and patients are aware of the diagnosis, they will inevitably fear for the future. This fear may make them very perceptive to unpleasant experiences and stimuli. It will considerably reduce anxiety when the nurse does not doubt what patients tell her about their pain experience. The nurse should convey that she believes them and is trying to understand how the patient experiences the pain (McCaffery and Moss, 1967).

Grief: This may be an emotional experience felt by those who lose a part of themselves through operation. The removal of a breast or the loss of a limb may be accompanied by feelings of great shock and sadness. The uncertain future may make self-control seem pointless, leading to a low pain-tolerance, emotional lability and feelings of resentment and fear.

Accident victims: Surgery resulting from accidents imposes special problems. There is almost always some increased anxiety caused by unexpectedly being in hospital.

For some the injury may be perceived as a minor irritation – the rugby football player who sustains a fractured femur during a heroic game is unlikely to see his accident as having a permanent effect on his life. However, many involved in traumatic injury requiring surgery are faced with the prospect of long-term uncertainty, loss of employment and perhaps litigation. These factors frequently serve to heighten awareness of pain later.

Additional discomforts
Pain resulting from the operation site may be aggravated by other factors. Observation and recognition of stimuli which might increase pain are vital if relief is to be appropriate and effective.

Technology: The development of surgical skills and medical technology have brought in its wake the widespread use of equipment which undoubtedly assists in the monitoring and safer treatment of patients who have undergone surgery. Patients who find themselves on the receiving end, however, may feel that staff give more attention to the equipment than to them. A nurse may check that the infusion pump is set correctly, look at the suction drain and glance at the observation chart, feeling that she has observed the patient when in fact she has observed everything except the patient. When equipment takes attention away from the patient, anxiety increases and may be reflected in a reduced tolerance for discomfort and in additional demands for pain-relief.

With the increasing use of technology, ward nurses frequently encounter equipment with which they are not familiar. This can produce problems for them because they are faced with something not immediately understood, and anxiety may be felt by the individual nurse. If she communicates this anxiety to the patient then he is likely to lose faith in her competence and ability. The remembered facial expression of a particular patient on parenteral feeding and intravenous antibiotics left a deep impression on the author (JH). This patient's distress was caused by a nurse, who, when changing the infusion, said to the patient that she did not know which way to turn the three-way tap. When nurses are faced with this sort of problem they must summon help without involving the patient in their dilemma.

Nausea: A degree of nausea and vomiting occurs in approximately one-third of postoperative patients. Vomiting may cause acute exacerbations of postoperative pain. The provision of a vomit bowl is obviously practical but does not provide much support for the vomiting patient. Physical contact and reassurance that the distress can be alleviated will always be appreciated. Often patients are afraid that the wound may burst, and assurance should be given that this is most unlikely. Instruction as to how the wound can be supported should be given pre-operatively (see Fig. 5/4, p.68). When a nasogastric tube is in situ, aspiration of stomach contents reduces vomiting. If the feeling of nausea still persists anti-emetic preparations are sometimes prescribed and may be very helpful.

Tiredness: Weakness and fatigue are a common experience among postoperative patients. Ensuring periods of rest without interference from visitors, doctors and paramedical staff is an important nursing role. Unrelieved fatigue can cause great distress and in turn aggravates, or induces, other problems, including an unwillingness to mobilise and breathe deeply.

A rest hour in the day during which time patients are not disturbed is much appreciated. Nurses should ensure that the patients are comfortable before the blinds are lowered. Pre-operative patients who do not want to rest should be asked to spend this quiet hour in the day room so that those requiring peace are able to achieve it.

Position: Increased pain is experienced when the patient's position in bed is uncomfortable. Physical support should go hand-in-hand with emotional care. An appropriate number of pillows placed where they are found to be of greatest value may provide more effective pain-relief than a specific pain-killer (Fig. 7/3). Whenever analgesia is given, the comfortable positioning of the patient at the same time should ensure the most effective overall pain-relief.

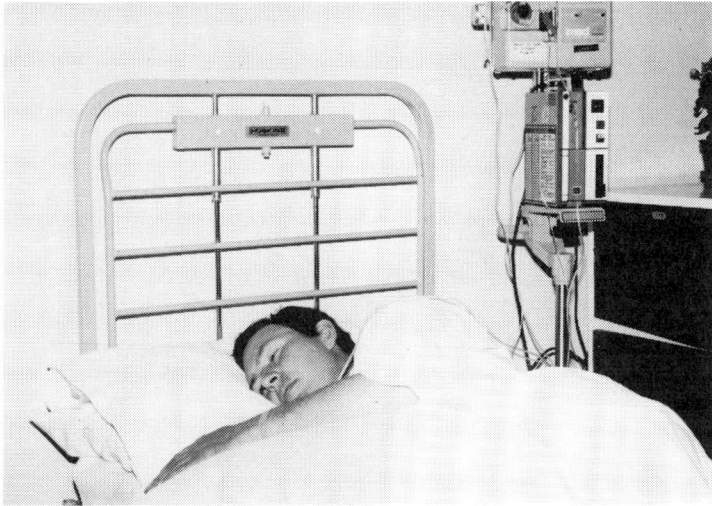

Fig. 7/3   Whenever analgesia is given the comfortable positioning of the patient should ensure the most effective overall pain relief

Dry mouth: Many find the problem of a dry mouth and sore throat very unpleasant after surgery. When oral fluids cannot be given, frequent oral toilet or mouthwashes should be offered. A gargle containing a gentle local anaesthetic may be prescribed to relieve sore throats resulting from the use of endotracheal tubes during anaesthesia. If allowed, ice cubes and sips of water should be offered.

Urinary retention: This is a relatively common problem affecting older men after surgery, and is due to benign prostatic hypertrophy obstructing the bladder. Lying in bed for a long time may lead to urinary retention on its own and one of the side-effects of some of the stronger narcotic analgesics is urinary retention. When it occurs, the patient may complain of both abdominal pain due to the distended bladder and additional wound pain caused by the distended abdomen.

The pain from a distended bladder is excruciating and may cause very great distress. It must be treated by somehow overcoming the obstruction, usually with a catheter. When the obstruction is relieved the pain will go immediately. It is important to question patients about their desire to pass urine and check that they do not have a distended bladder.

It is a disservice to give these patients analgesics, when what they need is relief of their obstruction.

In summary, the nurse has five major responsibilities in relation to analgesic medication for acute pain:

1. Assessment of the pain to determine whether, or not, the analgesic should be given, and, when.
2. Administration of an appropriate dose of prescribed analgesic, this may involve choosing the medication when more than one drug is prescribed.
3. Evaluation of the effectiveness of the analgesic following each administration.
4. Awareness of the possible side-effects of the analgesic.
5. Communication with medical staff to report promptly and accurately the need for a change in analgesic medication.

REFERENCE

McCaffery, M. and Moss, F. (1967). Nursing intervention for bodily pain. *American Journal of Nursing*, **67**, 1224–7.

BIBLIOGRAPHY

Copp, G. (1984). Nursing interventions in postoperative pain. *Nursing Mirror*, **159**, 13 (Theatre Nursing Special Supplement, VII-XV).

Drain, C. B. and Cain, R. S. (1981). The nursing implications of postoperative pain. *Military Medicine*, **146**, 127–31.

Hosking, J. (1985). Postoperative pain relief: nurses' knowledge and practice. *Nursing Mirror*, (Research Supplement), **160**, 5, ii–vi.

Sofaer, B. (1983). Pain relief – the importance of communication. *Nursing Times*, **79**, 49, 32–5.

Weis, O. et al (1983). Attitudes of patients, house staff and nurses toward postoperative analgesic care. *Anaesthetics and Analgesia*, **62**, 70–4.

Chapter Eight

ANALGESICS – EFFICACY AND CLASSIFICATION

ANALGESIC EFFICACY

All analgesics (pain-killers) show a 'dose-response effect'. In general, this means that when the dose of the drug is increased there is an increase in the analgesic effect; when the dose is decreased there is a decrease in effect. However, they do not show an unlimited increase in effect as the dose is continually raised (Fig. 8/1). Each analgesic has a maximum amount of effect, beyond which it will not go, no matter how much the dose is increased (Fig. 8/2). This maximum amount of analgesia is characteristic for each analgesic and is known as the analgesic 'efficacy'. Strong analgesics like morphine have a high efficacy which allows them to be used to treat the most severe pain when given in a big enough dose. On the other hand, weaker analgesics like codeine have a lower efficacy and cannot be used to treat very severe pain, even when given in very large doses. They can be used to treat moderate pain provided they are given in a suitable dose. Relatively weak analgesics such as paracetamol are only capable of treating relatively mild pain, because of their low efficacy.

Obviously a strong analgesic is capable of treating mild pain and requires only a small dose to do so. The aim should always be to use a drug with the lowest efficacy which will still successfully treat the patient's pain, because the reduction in efficacy tends to limit the severity of dose-dependent side-effects. In other words, patients with minor headaches should be treated with minor analgesics such as aspirin, not major ones like morphine because morphine would have the potential for much worse side-effects.

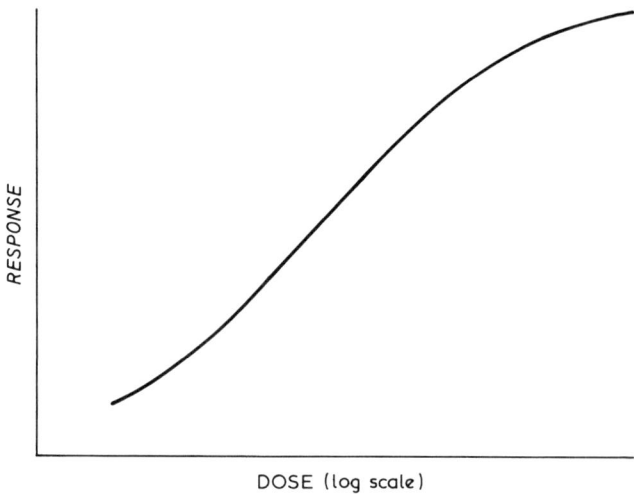

Fig. 8/1   A dose-response curve

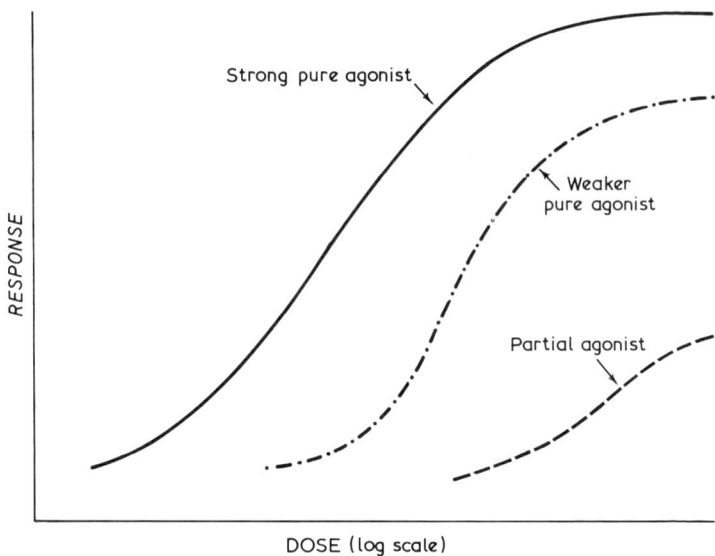

Fig. 8/2   Dose-response curves for 3 different types of analgesic

HOW TO CLASSIFY ANALGESICS

Analgesics may be classified as agonists, antagonists, partial agonist/partial antagonist, non-steroidal anti-inflammatory drugs (NSAID), and a mixed group of drugs which do not fit into any specific group.

Agonists

In Chapter 3 the concept of receptors, with reference to transmission of electrical impulses from one nerve to another, was discussed. It was shown that some transmitters had excitatory effects, while others were inhibitory. Many of the analgesics normally used in hospital are related to morphine and are called narcotics. The body produces a variety of transmitters which are involved in pain control. The analgesic narcotics appear to work by stimulating the same receptors as some of those transmitters involved in control of pain impulses. Narcotics which work by simply activating these receptors and stimulating pain relief, are called narcotic 'agonists', of which morphine, pethidine, fentanyl and codeine are all examples.

Antagonists

There are some drugs which have a relatively high affinity for the opiate receptors in the body, but have no intrinsic activity of their own. Given on their own, they appear to do nothing at all. However, if the patient had previously been given a narcotic with intrinsic activity, such as morphine, it would be displaced from the receptors by the drug with no activity of its own. The effects of the active narcotic would appear to be reduced by the diluting effect of the competing drug with no intrinsic activity. In this way a competitive 'antagonist', such as naloxone may be used to overcome the effects of an overdose of narcotics like pethidine or morphine. If given in sufficient quantities, a pure 'antagonist' such as naloxone will reverse all the effects of a conventional narcotic analgesic.

In some circumstances its use may be life-saving; but, as well as reversing respiratory depression, pupillary constriction and all the other side-effects of the narcotics, it will, just as quickly, also reverse the analgesic effects. The sudden revelation to the patient of his pain may be distressing and possibly cause severe hypertension.

Partial agonist/partial antagonist

Between the pure agonists and the pure antagonists, there is a group of drugs which have some of the properties of both groups. This is the partial agonist/partial antagonist group which includes pentazocine, buprenorphine, and nalbuphine. They all have some intrinsic activity and so are capable of causing both analgesia and respiratory depression when given in a large enough dose. They also have some antagonist properties, which allow them to reverse the effects of the pure agonist analgesics. For example, it is possible to reverse the respiratory depression of a strong pure agonist like fentanyl with a partial agonist/partial antagonist like pentazocine, while maintaining a state of analgesia, because of the analgesic properties of the pentazocine. If the dose of pentazocine used for this reversal is relatively high, then it will cause its own respiratory depression.

This effect of the partial agonist/partial antagonist is widely known, but rarely is it deliberately put to use, because of its own intrinsic potential for causing respiratory depression. This group of drugs may occasionally cause problems when they are given with strong, pure agonists (Fig. 8/3). If the patient has been taking the pure agonist for some time and a partial agonist/partial antagonist was added with the

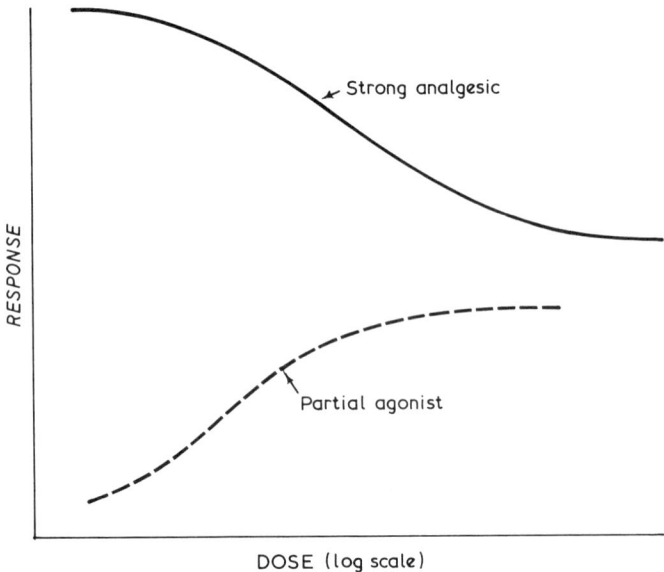

Fig. 8/3   Dose-response curve illustrating what happens when a partial agonist is added to a strong analgesic

aim of achieving additional analgesia, the quality of analgesia would actually become worse as the effects of the high efficacy analgesic were replaced by those of the partial agonist. The patient might also suffer the discomfort of an acute narcotic withdrawal syndrome as some of the narcotic effects were removed suddenly.

Non-steroidal anti-inflammatory drugs (NSAID)
This group reduces inflammation and, therefore, the amount of prostaglandin produced (see Chapter 3). Prostaglandin is known to sensitise pain receptors, so that by reducing the amount of it in an inflamed region the pain becomes less. These drugs act predominantly at the site of the painful stimulus rather than in the spinal cord or the brain, as the opiates do. This group includes, among others, aspirin, ibuprofen, ketoprofen, all of which have been advocated for the treatment of arthritic pain. These drugs have a relatively low efficacy when used to treat acute postoperative pain and so are appropriate only for mild pain. They come into their own when the pain is associated with inflammation and under such conditions may work better than the most potent narcotics.

Other analgesics
The last group of analgesic drugs which will be considered here is a small collection of drugs which are difficult to classify.

Volatile agents
Trilene and methoxyflurane are two such agents. They must be administered with a mask via a calibrated vapouriser (see Chapter 14). Nitrous oxide is a gaseous analgesic which also has to be delivered via a mask. As Entonox it is a mixture containing 50 per cent oxygen and 50 per cent nitrous oxide. These three agents all work centrally on the brain, though their precise mechanisms are not yet known. Each of them is absorbed through the patient's lungs and so can be delivered in a non-invasive way. They are all effective within about 5 minutes and cease to be so within a few minutes after stopping administration. This makes them very flexible for use when pain is intermittent or of short duration.

Ketamine
Ketamine is a powerful analgesic agent which must be given par-enterally. It does not appear to work at opiate receptors and has no effect on prostaglandin synthesis. Like the previous three agents it

may cause profound somnolence and anaesthesia if given in sufficient amounts. However, it does not appear to cause dose-dependent respiratory depression, as the opiates do, and yet is powerful enough to treat severe pain. Its main problem is a liability to cause sedation and hallucinations.

Local anaesthetics
The local anaesthetics could be considered a complete group in their own right, but they are included here for simplicity. Local anaesthetics, such as lignocaine and bupivacaine, act by stopping conduction of nervous impulses at the point where they are infiltrated. This means that local anaesthetics will stop all sensations travelling from the affected region; they will stop the motor impulses travelling to the affected part, so that the region becomes paralysed; and finally they will stop the autonomic impulses travelling to and from that region, so that there may be alterations in the blood flow to it. The size and position of the region affected will depend on which nerves have had impulses travelling in them stopped by the local anaesthetic. This in turn depends entirely on where the local anaesthetic has been put. It follows that to be effective, the local anaesthetic must be put in the correct place. Some surgeons and most anaesthetists will have been trained in the use of local anaesthetics in this way, but other members of staff are unlikely to have the experience and skill to use these drugs safely and effectively.

An exception to this general rule is the use of epidural catheters for labour pain, or severe thoracic and abdominal or back pain. In these instances a fine diameter epidural catheter is introduced into the epidural space (see Fig. 14/5, p. 137) of the patient by a doctor – usually an anaesthetist. The external (proximal) end of the catheter can then be secured in a convenient position to allow a nurse to inject the prescribed local anaesthetic down the catheter, knowing that the distal end of the catheter was placed in the epidural space by the doctor. Even so, midwives and nurses must be *trained* to perform the topping-up safely, and will have need to be certified as having achieved a satisfactory level of skill before being allowed to do this unsupervised (see Chapter 14).

Chapter Nine

THE MAJOR ANALGESICS

This group of drugs has the highest efficacy for relieving pain and they are capable of completely abolishing the most severe pain provided they are given in a large enough dose. Virtually all the drugs in this group are relatives of the opiate family of compounds. As previously indicated, they appear to work by substituting themselves at receptor sites in the brain and spinal cord instead of locally produced, short-acting molecules used to control pain impulses. Their high efficacy for analgesia does, however, carry with it an associated high risk of side-effects. In general, the effects of these drugs are a mixture of excitation and depression (see Chapter 12).

MORPHINE

Morphine is the standard major analgesic by which the rest are judged. It is the most important extract from opium, which is the milky exudate of the cut seed-head of the unripe poppy plant *Papaver somniferum*.

Metabolism

In man, morphine is well absorbed after intramuscular injection, but is much less potent when given orally. Blood from the small bowel carrying the absorbed morphine must all pass through the liver before getting into the systemic circulation. Approximately two-thirds of the oral dose is immediately metabolised by the normal liver, leaving only one-third to get into the systemic blood and have an effect. Morphine is also removed from the systemic blood as it goes through the liver. Most of the morphine is metabolised into inactive morphine glucuronide, which is then excreted in the urine. About 5 per cent of a parenterally given dose of morphine is excreted as the unchanged drug. Some excretion occurs in faeces, bile and other fluids such as saliva, perspiration and milk.

Dosage
The usual dose of morphine by intramuscular injection is between 10 and 15mg for a 70kg man. In this way analgesia for severe pain will usually last about 4 hours, while for moderate pain it may last a little longer. For much smaller or larger patients the dose may be adjusted on the basis that 0.15mg of intramuscular morphine be given for each kg of the patient's weight. The oral dose of morphine is usually three times the patient's intramuscular dose. It is almost impossible to predict an intravenous dose of morphine for a patient in advance. As with all the strong analgesics, it is normal practice to give the intravenous dose of the drug by slow titration of the drug against the individual patient's response to it.

Side-effects
Respiratory depression is the most important, and serious, side-effect, not only of morphine but also of the other strong opiate analgesics. This side-effect is dose-dependent and potentially life-threatening. When the drug is given orally or intramuscularly, doses which leave the patient with significant amounts of residual pain are unlikely to cause significant respiratory depression. When a patient is in severe pain which requires opiates like morphine in large doses to achieve good quality analgesia, these doses will cause some respiratory depression and consequently must be monitored carefully. As with the management of diabetes using insulin, so the management of severe pain requires careful monitoring not only of the effects of the therapy, but also the effects of the disease.

Constipation is associated with morphine administration. This fact is utilised in some diarrhoea mixtures such as Kaolin and Morphine Mixture BNF.

Spasm of smooth muscle in the sphincters can also be caused by morphine. This may affect the ciliary muscles of the eye leading to the pin-point pupils associated with morphine and other opiates. Biliary spasm and urinary retention are also examples of this effect by morphine on smooth muscle.

Sedation is a common side-effect of the major analgesics and morphine is no exception. Like respiratory depression, it is dose-dependent, but unlike respiratory depression it tends to occur at the same or, sometimes, at lower doses than those needed to treat severe pain. In doses used in clinical practice, sedation is very common and under some circumstances may be an advantage. However, it may lead to respiratory difficulties, particularly when patients are being nursed on their backs because transient obstruction of the airway may occur as the tongue falls backward due to gravity (Fig. 9/1). Heavy sedation

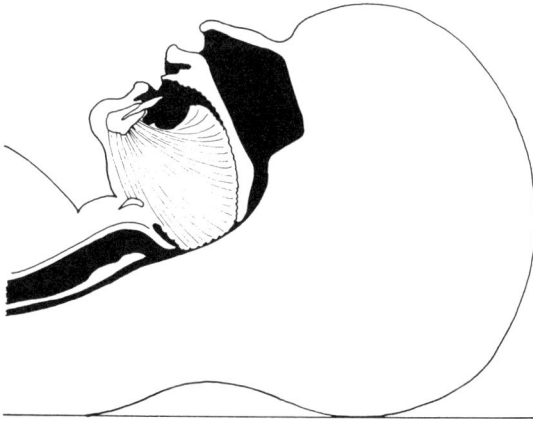

Fig. 9/1   A heavily sedated patient is at risk of airway obstruction due to the tongue falling back when lying supine

over several days with drugs like morphine may lead to pulmonary collapse, consolidation and infection; this is due to the patient's inability to participate actively in physiotherapy as well as spending long periods static in bed.

Histamine release
Morphine and some of the other opiates may release histamine, which in some individuals may cause itching in various parts of the body. It may lead to a localised 'weal and flare' reaction at the site of injection or along the vein if given intravenously. Rarely, the histamine released may trigger bronchospasm, particularly in asthmatics.

Tolerance

Patients on morphine for several days may develop tolerance to it, in that the dose required to produce a particular effect, such as adequate analgesia, may slowly increase. Such tolerance is simply a nuisance, as it merely needs a corresponding increase in the dose to keep the patient adequately treated.

Physical dependence to the morphine may develop after a week or more of regular treatment. When morphine is stopped after the treatment of acute pain, any resulting reaction is likely to be so mild as to be hardly noticed by the patient. However, if the effects of the morphine are abruptly terminated by the administration of either a partial agonist such as buprenorphine or nalbuphine, or a reversal agent such as naloxone, then the reaction will be more obvious. Such a reaction may include sweating, hyperventilation, diarrhoea and vomiting.

Like most of the other strong narcotic analgesics, morphine is capable of supporting both psychic and physical dependence. It therefore has the potential for abuse and its use and storage are strictly controlled in the United Kingdom by the Dangerous Drugs Act (see Chapter 15).

PETHIDINE

Pethidine is a synthetic narcotic analgesic, sometimes known as meperidine. It is one of the most widely prescribed potent analgesics and is commonly used for labour pain.

Metabolism

Pethidine is well absorbed by all routes of administration, although it is less reliable when given by mouth. Peak blood levels occur 1 to 2 hours after oral administration; after intravenous administration the blood levels peak within a minute or so and then fall rapidly over the next 2 hours. Given parenterally, 75mg of pethidine produces the same peak analgesia as 10mg of morphine, but, the duration of the action of pethidine is significantly shorter than that of the equivalent dose of morphine, so that injections need to be given more frequently.

Much of the popularity of pethidine for use in labour rested on early reports that it caused less respiratory depression in the neonate than other potent analgesics. Cambell et al (1961), however, showed that morphine and pethidine caused an equal amount of respiratory depression in the neonate. Pethidine crosses the placental barrier and can be detected in the urine of infants delivered from mothers who were given pethidine during labour. Once pethidine has found its way into the newborn infant, its effects last much longer than they would in a more mature individual, because the immature liver of the neonate is incapable of metabolising pethidine as quickly as an adult.

Very little pethidine is excreted unchanged: most of it is metabolised in the liver into a variety of compounds such as norpethidine, pethidinic acid and norpethidinic acid. Some of these breakdown products are active. The norpethidine produced in large amounts after a pethidine overdose probably accounts for some of the excitatory phenomena, such as hyperactive reflexes and convulsions. The breakdown products of pethidine are mostly conjugated in the liver and then excreted in the urine.

Side-effects
Pethidine produces most of the typical narcotic analgesic side-effects such as sedation, nausea and vomiting. Like morphine, it releases histamine, causes pupillary constriction and induces respiratory depression. Because of its structural similarity to atropine, pethidine may also possess some of the latter's properties. This could lead to a reduction in the incidence of biliary colic and possibly less constipation, although the evidence for this is conflicting.

PAPAVERETUM

Papaveretum (Omnopon) is widely prescribed in the United Kingdom for both anaesthetic premedication and postoperative pain. It is a standardised mixture made from an opium concentrate containing 50 per cent anhydrous morphine. The other 50 per cent contains the hydrochlorides of the remaining opium alkaloids, mainly thebaine, narcotine, papaverine and codeine. The codeine may increase its antitussive effect reducing the patient's urge to cough, while the papaverine acts as a smooth muscle relaxant and may worsen a postoperative ileus. Many clinicians believe that papaveretum causes fewer side-effects than an equivalent dose of morphine, but there is not good evidence to support this. On the other hand, there is evidence to show that the opium alkaloids mixed with the morphine of papaveretum tend to dilute its effect, making it less potent than the same dose of morphine given alone (Keeri-Santo, 1976). These other alkaloids also interfere with the clearance from the body of the morphine in papaveretum, making it shorter-acting than the same dose of morphine given alone.

Dosage

The usual dose of papaveretum is between 15 and 20mg for a fit 70kg patient. The dose is usually reduced for older patients as they are more sensitive to its effects and it is probably better not to prescribe it for the over-70s. Papaveretum may be given orally, subcutaneously, intramuscularly or intravenously. Weight for weight, 20mg of papaveretum contains approximately 13.5mg of morphine as the sulphate or hydrochloride – the forms usually prescribed. However, the diluting effect of the other alkaloids in it reduce its effect to the equivalent of that of about 10mg of morphine sulphate or hydrochloride.

DIAMORPHINE (HEROIN)

Diamorphine is the diacetyl analogue of morphine and because of this it is approximately twice as powerful. The usual dose is between 5 and 10mg, given subcutaneously. Continued use causes tolerance and consequently it may be necessary to give it in much larger doses where patients have been using it for several days or even weeks. Its duration of effect is less than that of morphine and may be only 2 to 4 hours. It may cause less nausea, vomiting and constipation than morphine. It may also cause less sedation and more euphoria than morphine. Dundee, Clarke and Loan (1967) observed that it appeared to cause an increase in sedation compared with morphine without any increase in euphoria or anxiolysis. On the other hand, there is no doubt about its ability to induce addiction. Because of this its manufacture is forbidden in the United States and many other countries. In the United Kingdom its use is reserved for patients with terminal illnesses, in whom the problem of addiction is irrelevant.

FENTANYL

This is a synthetic narcotic, related to pethidine. It may be given intravenously, intramuscularly, epidurally or orally, but is usually given intravenously, when it has a much shorter duration of action than an equipotent dose of pethidine. Morrison et al (1971) estimated that 0.2mg of fentanyl was equipotent with 10mg of morphine.

Intravenous fentanyl given in doses greater than this were liable to cause increasing respiratory depression.

During surgery doses of 0.2mg are often given every 20 to 30 minutes. Larger doses than this have a more prolonged duration.

Fentanyl has a high analgesic efficacy and causes little sedation when used for postoperative pain. Its short duration makes it more suitable for use by continuous intravenous or epidural infusion than by intermittent bolus injections.

REFERENCES

Cambell, C., Phillips, C. C. and Frazier, T. M. (1961). Analgesia during labour: a comparison of pentobarbital, meperidine and morphine. *Obstetrics and Gynaecology*, **17**, 714–18.

Dundee, J. W., Clarke, R. S. J. and Loan, W. B. (1967). Comparative toxicity of diamorphine, morphine and methadone. *Lancet*, **2**, 221.

Keeri-Santo, M. (1976). Papaveretum for anaesthesia and its comparison with morphine. Anaesthetic time/dose curves. *Journal of the Canadian Anaesthetics Society*, **23**, 239–43.

Morrison, J. D., Loan, W. B. and Dundee, J. W. (1971). Controlled comparison of the efficacy of fourteen preparations in the relief of postoperative pain. *British Medical Journal*, **3**, 287.

Chapter Ten

RESPIRATORY STIMULANTS

One of the major side-effects of potent narcotic analgesia is respiratory depression. Patients who are most at risk to this problem may be the same as those who are in the greatest need of potent analgesia, for example grossly obese patients, those with chronic chest disease or who are debilitated. They are the patients most at risk to drug-induced respiratory depression, yet they will all recover better from surgery if they can be kept reasonably pain-free.

There are three groups of drugs available which will increase respiration under the above circumstances:

1. Narcotic antagonists, e.g. naloxone.
2. Partial agonist/partial antagonists.
3. Central stimulants, e.g. doxapram.

NALOXONE

The narcotic antagonists include the pure antagonist naloxone which in clinical doses appears to have no additional effects of its own, but will reverse all the effects of narcotic agonists such as morphine, if given in a large enough dose. The usual dose-range of naloxone for adults is between 0.2 and 0.8mg intravenously or intramuscularly. The intravenous dose is unlikely to last more than 20 to 30 minutes, which may be less than the duration of the underlying respiratory depression. If this is the case, then a second period of respiratory depression may appear, some time after the first, and a second dose of the antagonist will need to be given. Unfortunately, naloxone will reverse *all* the effects of the narcotic analgesics, not simply the respiratory depression and somnolence; pain is therefore likely to reappear. No further dose of the narcotic can be given at this stage because the patient must have had too much previously to cause the respiratory depression.

PARTIAL AGONIST/PARTIAL ANTAGONISTS

This group of drugs, which includes pentazocine, buprenorphine and nalbuphine, is capable of partially reversing the effects of agonist narcotics such as morphine and pethidine. This effect is 'double-edged', for while such drugs have the advantage of not leaving the patient without pain-relief at all, as naloxone would do, they will substitute their own side-effects instead. These side-effects may include respiratory depression.

Two partial agonist/partial antagonists of the narcotics are discussed largely for historical reasons, and also because in some hospitals, particularly on obstetric units, they may still be in use. They are nalorphine and levallorphan. Both drugs have weak analgesic properties; levallorphan being slightly more analgesic than nalorphine. Both are capable of antagonising the respiratory depressant effects of pure narcotic agonists such as pethidine. However, they do cause respiratory depression, and if given to patients who have not actually got *narcotic*-induced respiratory depression, will make that depression worse. For many years nalorphine and levallorphan have been used in obstetric units to counter the effects of pethidine and other narcotic analgesics given to mothers in labour. If they were not given, the narcotics would cause respiratory depression in the newborn babies.

Dosage

The dose of nalorphine is between 3 and 5mg intravenously to the mother, or 0.2 to 0.5mg given into the umbilical vein of the baby. The dose of levallorphan is between 1 and 2mg intravenously to the mother or 0.25mg given into the umbilical vein of the newborn baby. Both drugs have been almost totally superseded by naloxone.

DOXAPRAM

Doxapram hydrochloride is the most widely used of the central stimulant group of drugs. It acts directly on the respiratory centre to stimulate respiration. In low doses it will cause an increase in the depth of respiration only, but if the dose is increased there will also be an increase in the rate of breathing. These effects are usually accompanied by an increase in the heart rate and rise of blood pressure. In overdosage there may be a marked tachycardia, high blood pressure, vomiting, apprehension and, eventually, convulsions. Unlike naloxone, doxapram appears to have no effect upon the analgesia of narcotics.

Dosage
Doxapram can be given by bolus intravenous injections of 1.0 to 1.5mg/kg body-weight every 1 to 2 hours, or by continuous intravenous infusion of 1.5 to 3.0mg/minute for as long as required. The drug is rapidly metabolised and does not accumulate if given in this way. Because of its effects upon the heart and blood pressure, doxapram should be avoided in patients with severe hypertension, thyrotoxicosis or ischaemic heart disease. It should be used with caution in epileptics. Its actions are potentiated in patients taking monoamine-oxidase inhibitors.

Chapter Eleven

MODERATE AND MINOR ANALGESICS AND LOCAL ANAESTHETICS

MODERATE ANALGESICS

The moderate analgesics are those drugs with less analgesic efficacy than the major analgesics. They are capable of treating moderate pain, but are not successful in controlling severe pain. The group includes some of the pure agonist narcotics with reduced efficacy, most of the partial agonist/partial antagonist analgesics, and some other agents which are difficult to classify.

Codeine

Codeine is a naturally-occurring narcotic found in opium. Structurally it is related to morphine and is made commercially from morphine. It may be given orally as tablets or linctus, and is well absorbed by this route. The oral:parenteral potency ratio is two-thirds, which is unusually high for a narcotic.

Metabolism

In the liver codeine is metabolised into morphine and norcodeine, which are then excreted, with codeine, almost entirely in the urine. Up to 86 per cent of a dose of codeine will have appeared in the urine in some form during the 24 hours after administration. About half will appear as free or conjugated codeine, about 10 per cent will appear as free or conjugated morphine and approximately 20 per cent will appear as free or conjugated norcodeine. Only traces will appear in the faeces.

Dosage
The usual dose is between 10 and 60mg. Codeine may be given intramuscularly in doses of up to 60mg, though further increases in this dose will lead only to increased side-effects, such as restlessness or respiratory depression rather than an increase in pain relief.

Side-effects
Side-effects of codeine include constipation, nausea, vertigo, sedation and respiratory depression, though all of these, apart from the constipation, are less of a problem than with morphine. Because of its potent constipating effect, codeine is widely used in anti-diarrhoea mixtures. Codeine reduces the irritability of the respiratory tract and is used as an antitussive agent to prevent troublesome, unproductive coughing. As with the other narcotic analgesics tolerance may occur to codeine when it is given continuously for a long time. Dependence on the effects of codeine may also occur if it is given for long periods, but the incidence is very low. The dependence liability of codeine is far lower than that of morphine or the other more powerful narcotic analgesics.

Codeine has an analgesic efficacy similar to that of aspirin. It is often found in commercial mixtures with other analgesics such as aspirin or paracetamol.

Dihydrocodeine
This is probably the most widely prescribed of this group of drugs. It is related to codeine but is slightly more potent.

Dosage
Dihydrocodeine may be given orally in doses of 30 to 60mg; intramuscularly in doses of 25 to 50mg; or intravenously by titration against effect.

Side-effects
Dihydrocodeine is a strong cough suppressant and was produced originally for this effect. It also causes marked constipation and a degree of nausea and vertigo. When given orally or intramuscularly its duration of analgesia is about 3 hours. Although 60mg of dihydrocodeine given intravenously is almost as analgesic as 10mg of morphine, at this dose level it does cause significant respiratory depression and further increases in dose will result in little additional analgesia but a

significant increase in side-effects. Dihydrocodeine may cause narcotic dependence, but most addicts would consider it a very poor substitute for morphine. The dependence-liability of dihydrocodeine is about the same as that of codeine.

PARTIAL AGONISTS/PARTIAL ANTAGONISTS

Pentazocine
Pentazocine is a synthetic narcotic with analgesic properties. It was produced during a search for a narcotic antagonist. It has the ability to cause analgesia and respiratory depression, while also being able to reverse some of these effects in other narcotic analgesics.

Metabolism
Only 2 to 12 per cent of a dose of pentazocine is likely to be excreted unchanged, the rest being metabolised before excretion. The majority of excretion is from the kidneys and the major metabolite is conjugated pentazocine.

Dosage
It may be given orally in doses of 25 to 100mg; by subcutaneous or intramuscular injection in doses of 30 to 60mg; and intravenously by titration against effect. Following oral administration, peak plasma levels occur after 1 to 3 hours, whereas after intramuscular injection peak plasma levels occur 15 to 20 minutes after injection. The oral:parenteral potency ratio is approximately one-third and absorption of the oral dose may be quite erratic; 30mg of intramuscular pentazocine provides about the same amount of analgesia as 50 to 100mg of pethidine given intramuscularly and lasts for almost the same amount of time, i.e. 3 to 4 hours. Pentazocine is capable of crossing the placental barrier, but appears to do so more slowly than pethidine.

Side-effects
Pentazocine causes similar side-effects to morphine, with a few exceptions. It causes respiratory depression of similar severity to an equi-analgesic dose of morphine and may cause nausea, vomiting and sedation as well. Unlike morphine, parenteral pentazocine is associated with a rise in blood pressure which is thought to be due to the release of catecholamines. It is also associated with a relatively high incidence of

vivid dreams and hallucinations. Drug dependence has been reported with pentazocine, but this is unusual and the drug generally has a low abuse potential. Pentazocine has quite strong antagonist properties and in the past has been used to antagonise the effects of narcotic analgesics given during surgery. However, during the early post-operative period, because of its inherent respiratory depression, this technique of using it for deliberate narcotic reversal while maintaining analgesia is little used now.

Buprenorphine
Buprenorphine is a semi-synthetic opioid analgesic, related to thebaine. It appears to be approximately 30 times as potent as morphine when given parenterally.

Metabolism
When given orally (by tablet) the drug is almost entirely metabolised by the liver before having a systemic effect. However, it is rapidly absorbed by the mucosa of the tongue over 10 minutes and then slowly released into the blood during the next 4 to 5 hours. There is usually a delay of about 2 hours between the administration of sublingual tablets and the onset of analgesia because the drug remains fixed in the buccal mucosa during this period. Because of this delay, it is unwise to give sublingual buprenorphine only when the patient demands it for pain relief.

Up to 70 per cent of a dose will be excreted in the faeces with the rest being excreted by the kidneys. Virtually all of it is conjugated in the liver into glucuronides which are inactive and then excreted in the bile. Buprenorphine is excreted in the breast milk of lactating women, but the drug is likely to be present only as a very small dose which, as has already been stated, will be almost entirely metabolised in the infant's gut wall and liver before having systemic effects.

Dosage
Doses of 0.3 to 0.6mg intramuscularly or intravenously, or 0.2 to 0.4mg sublingually may be given. The drug lasts between 6 and 8 hours by either route. Approximately 50 per cent of the sublingual dose appears to be systemically available, giving a sublingual:parenteral potency ratio of one half.

Side-effects
Buprenorphine's main side-effects include sedation, nausea and vomiting. The latter two are more prominent in ambulant patients. Buprenorphine 0.3mg and morphine 12.5mg, both given intramuscularly, have been shown to give the same degree of respiratory depression. Unlike other more conventional narcotics, the actions of buprenorphine may be quite difficult to reverse with naloxone because buprenorphine has a very high affinity for the opiate receptors and will stick to them firmly. Respiratory stimulants such as doxapram, have been successfully used in patients with buprenorphine-induced respiratory depression. Buprenorphine appears to be relatively free of psychic effects, causing neither euphoria or dysphoria. It appears to have a very low addiction liability.

Nalbuphine

Nalbuphine is another semi-synthetic opioid analgesic with partial agonist/partial antagonist properties. Structurally it is related to both the antagonist naloxone and the potent opioid analgesic oxymorphone.

Metabolism
Unlike most of the other opiate-type analgesics, nalbuphine's major route of excretion is faecal, with less than 26 per cent being excreted in the urine.

Dosage
Doses of 10 to 20mg can be given intravenously or intramuscularly. These doses appear to provide analgesia equivalent to that achieved with 5 to 8mg of morphine and last for about 4 hours. When given intravenously nalbuphine appears to reach its peak effect 20 to 25 minutes after injection. At present there is no oral version available. Its predicted oral:parenteral potency ratio is one-quarter; on that basis the oral dose would be approximately four times that of the parenteral.

Side-effects
Its major side-effect appears to be sedation, though it may also cause some nausea, vomiting, dry mouth and sweating. It appears to be relatively free from psychic effects such as dysphoria and euphoria and so has a very low abuse potential. It is, however, a *very* potent antagonist of morphine-like agonists and may precipitate an acute

abstinence syndrome in patients who have been taking these drugs regularly.

Nefopam

Nefopam is a non-narcotic analgesic, which is structurally unrelated to any of the other analgesics. It is not bound to narcotic receptors and so does not interfere with the actions of narcotic analgesics which the patients may also be taking. The mode of action of nefopam is obscure and its nearest structural relatives are the anti-histamine diphenhydramine and the anti-parkinson drug orphenadrine. Nefopam shares none of the features of these two drugs at all, apart from their structural similarities.

Metabolism

The majority of nefopam is metabolised in the liver, with less than 5 per cent being excreted unchanged in the urine. Almost 90 per cent of administered nefopam appears in the urine as metabolites, with most of the rest appearing in faeces.

Dosage

The oral dose of nefopam is between 30 and 60mg and may be given 3 to 4 times daily; the intramuscular dose is 20mg which may be given 4- to 6-hourly; and the intravenous dose is usually between 10 and 20mg, given by titration against effect. Nefopam has a pronounced 'ceiling-effect', which limits its analgesia to the equivalent of that obtained with 50mg of pethidine or 5mg of morphine, because of its relatively low analgesic efficacy.

Side-effects

Its major side-effects are nausea, vomiting, sweating, flushing and tachycardia. It may cause a little pain at the site of injection. The major disadvantage of nefopam is probably its low efficacy. It is one of the lowest in the moderate analgesic group as a whole, making it quite unsatisfactory for severe pain.

The major advantages of nefopam appear to be its relative lack of sedation, compared with some of the other moderately potent analgesics, and its relatively low level of respiratory depression.

THE MINOR ANALGESICS

The antipyretic anti-inflammatory analgesics

Acetylsalicylic acid was first prepared in 1853 and first used clinically in 1899 to treat patients with rheumatic diseases. It has antipyretic, anti-inflammatory and analgesic properties and is a typical member of a group of compounds called the antipyretic, anti-inflammatory analgesics. These drugs are particularly useful for the treatment of headache, rheumatic and muscular pain, arthritic pain and pain arising from connective tissue. The antipyretic and anti-inflammatory properties of the individual members of this group are not always found in similar proportions, so that some are hardly antipyretic at all, while others may have very little anti-inflammatory property.

The anti-inflammatory action of these drugs is thought to be due to their selective inhibition of an enzyme called prostaglandin synthetase, which is essential for the production of prostaglandin. Prostaglandin, which is released at sites of inflammation, sensitises tissues to the effects of bradykinin, histamine and 5-hydroxytryptamine – all agents which cause pain and inflammation. The anti-inflammatory analgesics, such as aspirin, therefore appear to work by inhibiting production of one group of compounds, the prostaglandins, which if released will make inflammation worse and more painful.

Aspirin

Aspirin (acetylsalicylic acid) is the standard antipyretic analgesic by which all the others are judged. It is administered orally, and is well absorbed from both the stomach and intestine.

Metabolism

The aspirin is rapidly hydrolysed in the intestine and circulation in to salicylic acid, which is rapidly redistributed to body tissues such as the kidney, liver, heart and lungs. It can cross the placental barrier, and is secreted in saliva, milk and bile. Salicylate is excreted in the urine, particularly when the urine is alkaline, when as much as 90 per cent will be excreted in the free form. However, when the urine is acid almost all the salicylate is conjugated in the liver with glycuronic acid or glycine.

Dosage

The official dose of aspirin is between 300mg and 1g. Adults are usually given 600mg in tablet form, when required, and repeated at 4-hourly intervals, when necessary. Aspirin has a very narrow therapeutic dose range. Below the correct dose, it has little or no effect, while above that dose there is virtually no increase in analgesia, only an increase in side-effects.

Effects
The antipyretic effects of aspirin are thought to be mediated by the hypothalamus, which causes an increase in sweating and hyperaemia of the skin. It also stimulates metabolism, increasing heat production. Normally this effect is masked by the cooling effects; however, if the patient cannot sweat because of fluid depletion, or the aspirin is given in overdose, then a hyperpyrexia may result.

Aspirin is a common cause of bleeding from gastric erosions. About 80 per cent of patients taking 4g or more per day will lose between 3 and 10ml of blood per day from chronic gastric bleeding. In some patients this may lead to an iron deficiency anaemia. Rarely, aspirin ingestion is the cause of massive gastro-intestinal bleeding. Bleeding is caused by an inhibition of platelet aggregation; if the doses are high and maintained for several days or weeks, a prolongation of the prothrombin time will occur.

Ibuprofen
Ibuprofen is a mild analgesic, antipyretic and anti-inflammatory agent, whose actions compare favourably with those of aspirin. It is rapidly absorbed when given by mouth and is metabolised to inactive products which are excreted from the kidneys. Initially, it is usually given in doses of 300mg 4 times daily, then reduced to 200mg 3 to 4 times daily. It is comparatively free from side-effects but occasionally causes dyspepsia, malaise and rashes.

KETAMINE

Ketamine hydrochloride is supplied as a clear liquid in multi-dose ampoules, containing 10, 50 or 100mg/ml of ketamine. It is a powerful analgesic *and* hypnotic agent, being used for the induction of anaesthesia. Doses of 10 to 50 micrograms/kg body-weight/minute may be infused to produce a state of analgesia, strong enough to carry out burns' dressings or even minor surgery. However, doses of 2mg/kg body-weight given intravenously or 10mg/kg body-weight intramuscularly may produce a state of unconsciousness.

Because of its liability to produce a state of unconsciousness, ketamine is usually only administered by trained anaesthetists. It has two major disadvantages: (1) a liability to cause drowsiness lasting for several hours after administration; and (2) it causes a high incidence of vivid dreams, some of which may be unpleasant, even progressing to frank hallucinations. Prior treatment with a drug such as lorazepam may markedly reduce the incidence of these dreams, but will increase the drowsiness. If patients are allowed to sleep quietly in a darkened room for some hours after the administration of ketamine, this appears to reduce the incidence of both dreaming and hallucinations.

Ketamine does not usually cause respiratory depression. Even when deeply asleep under ketamine anaesthesia, patients can usually maintain a patent upper airway, and both laryngeal and pharyngeal reflexes are present. It needs to be remembered that these factors are not absolute and patients can react differently. Constant monitoring is essential by the nurse. The administration of ketamine is associated with tachycardia and an increase in blood pressure. It is therefore particularly useful for those patients who may be at risk to hypotension, and for providing potent analgesia in difficult environments, such as at car crashes or other accidents where the victims may be trapped and in pain.

LOCAL ANAESTHETICS

These are drugs which can penetrate nerve fibres and stop nerve impulses from being conducted in those parts affected by the local anaesthetic. In general, small diameter fibres are the most susceptible to their effects. Therefore at very low concentrations local anaesthetics will only affect fine diameter autonomic nerves, causing vasodilation and dry skin in the affected area. As the concentration of the drug is increased, the larger nerve fibres will be affected. The pain fibres will be affected first, followed by those which conduct other sensory modalities; the motor fibres which send impulses to the muscles causing them to contract are affected last. Pain from an operation, or wound, can therefore be stopped in its pathway to the spinal cord and brain by applying local anaesthetic to the nerves carrying that painful sensation.

Side-effects

Following local anaesthetic nerve blocking there will probably be loss of all sensation in the affected region. There may also be paralysis of muscles supplied by the motor nerves affected, and vasodilation which, if extensive, may lead to a fall in blood pressure. But, by blocking *all* nerve conduction from the painful region, local anaesthetics are capable of providing *total* loss of the sensation of pain.

Two local anaesthetics which are widely used in the United Kingdom are lignocaine and bupivacaine. Their onset, time and duration of effect depend to some extent on the way they are given and the regions into which they are used. Lignocaine usually lasts about 1 to 2 hours, while bupivacaine lasts 2 to 4 hours. These times relate to the loss of sensation, the actual *pain* relief obtained may be much longer lasting.

Administration

There are a variety of techniques available for the relief of acute pain using local anaesthetics, all of which require a degree of technical expertise normally associated with anaesthetists. Consequently it is the anaesthetist who usually initiates postoperative pain therapy using local anaesthetics. Most techniques use a single dose of the local anaesthetic, which is then allowed to wear off, after which the patient may start alternative analgesic treatment. Some techniques require the insertion of a fine diameter plastic catheter into the region where the nerves are to be 'blocked'. Repeated doses of the local anaesthetic may then be given down the catheter as required. Epidural catheters may be inserted into the epidural space (see Fig. 14/5, p. 137). Repeated doses of local anaesthetic given through the catheter may be used to block all painful sensations coming from the lower abdomen, pelvis and lower limbs. In this way the pain of labour may be alleviated. This technique is also used for surgery on the lower limbs or pelvic organs and allows the provision of pain relief afterwards with repeated injections of the local anaesthetic. Epidural 'top-ups' are commonly performed in hospitals by nurses and midwives who have been specifically trained and certificated.

Nursing care

When nursing patients who have been given a local anaesthetic, great care should be taken of those parts of the body affected by the numbness, as the patient may damage it inadvertently. If the affected parts are paralysed, help should be given when the patient needs to move. The affected regions may be vasodilated which may cause postural hypotension, so care should be taken when sitting patients up after extensive local anaesthetic blocks.

Chapter Twelve

SUMMARY OF ANALGESICS IN COMMON USE FOR POSTOPERATIVE PAIN

DRUG	ADVANTAGES	DISADVANTAGES
Major analgesics		
morphine	High efficacy Well known Can be given orally Completely reversed by naloxone	Respiratory depression Nausea and sedation Tolerance A controlled drug

pethidine	High efficacy
	Well known
	Can be given orally
	Completely reversed
	  by naloxone
	May be used for
	  biliary colic
		Respiratory depression
		Nausea and sedation
		Tolerance
		A controlled drug
		Short acting

papaveretum (Omnopon)	High efficacy Well known Completely reversed by naloxone	Respiratory depression Nausea and sedation Tolerance A controlled drug Short acting A mixture

DRUG	ADVANTAGES	DISADVANTAGES
diamorphine (heroin)	High efficacy Well known Completely reversed by naloxone	Respiratory depression Nausea and sedation Tolerance A controlled drug Short acting Addiction potential
fentanyl	High efficacy Completely reversed by naloxone Little sedation	Respiratory depression Nausea A controlled drug Very short acting Usually given by infusion

Moderate analgesics

codeine	Little respiratory depression May be given orally	Only moderate efficacy Constipation Antitussive
dihydrocodeine	Higher efficacy than codeine May be given orally	More respiratory depression than codeine Constipation Antitussive
pentazocine	Moderately high efficacy May be given orally Low abuse potential May be given in labour	Respiratory depression Nausea and sedation Hallucinations Reverses other narcotics
buprenorphine	Moderately high efficacy May be given sublingually Low abuse potential Long acting	Respiratory depression Nausea and sedation Reverses other narcotics Slow onset Poor reversal by naloxone
nalbuphine	Low abuse potential No psychic effects Little nausea	Respiratory depression Only moderate efficacy Sedation Strongly reverses other narcotics No oral version

DRUG	ADVANTAGES	DISADVANTAGES
nefopam	Respiratory depression unlikely Lack of sedation May be given orally	Only moderate efficacy Nausea Sweating and tachycardia

Non-steroidal anti-inflammatory drugs (NSAIDs)

DRUG	ADVANTAGES	DISADVANTAGES
aspirin	Anti-inflammatory No respiratory depression Antipyretic No interactions with narcotics	Causes gastro-intestinal bleeding Low efficacy
paracetamol	No respiratory depression Antipyretic No interactions with narcotics	Low efficacy No anti-inflammatory action
ibuprofen, ketoprofen, fenoprofen	No respiratory depression Anti-inflammatory Antipyretic Less gastro-intestinal bleeding than with aspirin No interactions with narcotics	Low efficacy
naproxen	Slightly higher efficacy than the above group Fewer side-effects than the above group	

DRUG	ADVANTAGES	DISADVANTAGES
Others		
ketamine	High efficacy Respiration depression unusual Useful in potentially shocked patients Useful in difficult environments	Prolonged sedation Hallucinations Can only be given under anaesthetic supervision Not well known by staff
trilene, methoxyflurane, Entonox	Moderate efficacy Non-invasive route Relatively quick onset	Causes sedation Special equipment needed Not well known by staff Smells/pollution risk Entonox may be in cylinders
local anaesthetics, e.g. lignocaine, bupivacaine	Can stop all pain Can be of long duration No dose-dependent respiratory depression No sedation	Also stops all other sensations Causes paralysis of the affected region Special medical training required to perform the nerve blocks Invasive

Chapter Thirteen

REGIMES FOR ADMINISTERING ANALGESICS

The effectiveness of drugs for acute pain can be affected by the route of administration as well as by the actual regime. Chapter 14 will consider the routes of administration, while this chapter concentrates on the actual regimes, discussing the objectives, advantages and disadvantages of each.

As already discussed (see p. 78) there is considerable variation between different patients' responses to what appears to be the same surgical stimulus. Nevertheless, there is a general pattern to post-surgical pain which does apply to most patients (Fig. 13/1). The pain is usually at its worst in the immediate hours postoperatively, after

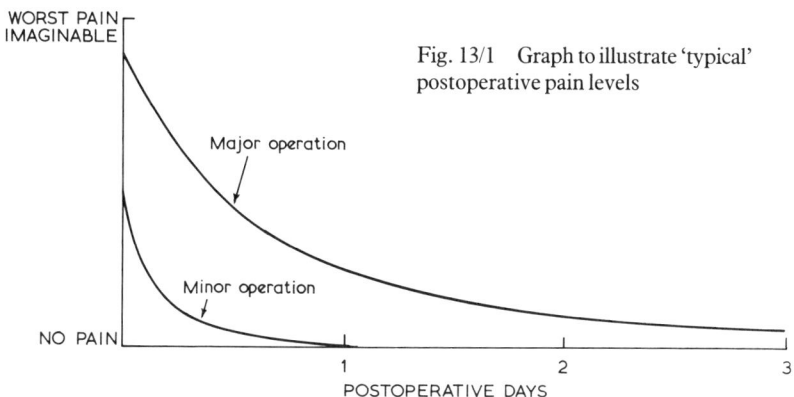

Fig. 13/1   Graph to illustrate 'typical' postoperative pain levels

which it declines over the remaining 24 hours. Depending upon the actual operation, it may take up to a week for the pain to go completely. During this time, patients often complain that movement of the scar hurts, but that while lying still they experience little or no pain.

An 'ideal' drug regime for acute pain should be able to provide analgesia of rapid onset when the patient requires it, in amounts which are appropriate for the particular patient and for his type of pain. The regime should be able to take account not only of increases, but also of decreases in the actual requirements for analgesia, and to do so safely. The ideal analgesic regime should be simple to use, unambiguous and not likely to generate administrative confusion. The ideal regime will, hopefully, not take up large amounts of nursing or medical time for its administration so that it may be judged cost-effective.

There are four basic regimes:

1. Single dose.
2. Repeated doses: (a) regular or (b) 'as required'.
3. Continuous administration.
4. Combinations of repeated doses and continuous administration.

THE SINGLE DOSE REGIME

This regime usually applies to the use of a local anaesthetic, the best example of which is the local anaesthetic injected into a patient's gum before commencing dental treatment. A single dose of local anaesthetic will block all sensation from the affected region not only during the procedure itself but also for several hours afterwards. The patient therefore feels no pain at all during the period when one would expect the pain to be at its worse. By the time the local anaesthetic wears off, the pain should have subsided sufficiently making the need for further analgesics either unnecessary, or only mild oral analgesics for a short time.

As a regional block, local anaesthetics may be used for a variety of surgical procedures, from minor peripheral surgery, to major operations such as caesarean section, hysterectomy and amputation. In each case the pain during the early postoperative period may be completely blocked by a single dose of local anaesthetic given as a spinal, epidural or nerve blocking injection. The disadvantage of this regime is that the patient's pain may continue to be severe once the local anaesthetic wears off; the regime will have stopped the pain only during the first postoperative hours when it was at its worst. The single dose of local anaesthetic is not usually repeated, because it requires an anaesthetist to administer it under sterile conditions.

If the patient is having minor surgery, the postoperative pain may only be moderate, in which case, a single dose of analgesic given during surgery, or soon afterwards, may be all that is required. The drug will have its peak effect at the same time as the patient is experiencing the worst pain, and the hope is that the effects will wear off at the same rate as the pain.

REPEATED DOSES

If the pain lasts longer than the analgesia achieved by a single dose of analgesic, then the dose may need to be repeated several times. This raises the question of how to decide when each subsequent dose should be given. There are two ways of doing this – regularly, or on-demand.

Regular

Previous chapters have discussed the variability between patients, in terms of the degree of pain they suffer and the amount of analgesic they require after similar operations. Nevertheless, when dealing with fit young patients having routine surgery, it is possible to make some generalisations about the doses of analgesics (and their likely duration) which will probably be required. If each of the repeated doses of analgesic is given just as the previous dose is expected to wear off, then one would hope that the patient would have no pain at all between each dose (Fig. 13/2). This type of regime has two main advantages:

1. The possibility of no periods without analgesia during the post-operative period, and
2. Planned administration of drugs during the postoperative period, allowing the nursing staff to anticipate and arrange for the staff required to give the drugs.

The two main disadvantages of this type of regime are:

1. There is no 'feedback' from the patients with these fixed regimes, so that if an inappropriate dose or time interval is used, the mistake may be repeated to the detriment of the patient.

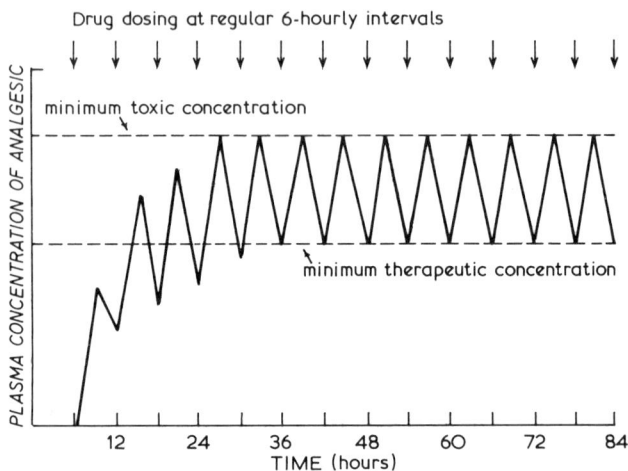

Fig. 13/2 Blood levels with fixed, regular doses of analgesic

2. Several patients may be written up for this type of regime to start immediately after operation. As the individual's surgery will finish at different times, the prescriptions will almost certainly be at different times. Such a regime can be difficult for nursing staff because each prescription will be out of phase with the next.

Drugs which have a delayed onset of analgesia are best given on a regular basis, for if they are given only when the patient has pain, there will be a delay after administration before the patient gains relief from his pain. Sublingual buprenorphine may take up to 2 hours before analgesia starts and so is best given regularly.

'As-required'
In the United Kingdom the commonest type of regime used for postoperative pain is the 'as-required by the patient', or 'prn' regime. This regime usually has a fixed dose of drug, but varies the dose-intervals. The assumption is that when a dose of analgesic starts to wear off, the patient will ask for another dose, which will start to work very soon afterwards. This regime tries to make allowances for the variability in duration of analgesics given to different patients. It also ensures that there is little or no accumulation of analgesic, as each dose is allowed to wear off before the next is given.

In theory this regime offers the patient flexibility to have more analgesia when he needs it, without the worry of getting too much.

In practice this regime appears to perform rather poorly. Patients tend to wait until their pain is unbearable before they ask for help, and nurses are then not always immediately available to respond. There may not be a qualified nurse available; the nurse may feel that the patient 'does not really have much pain', or has not waited long enough since the previous dose was given. Both patients and nurses may create delays with this type of regime, which can then result in poor quality analgesia resulting in long periods when there is no effective relief of pain.

Plasma concentration

As a rule, centrally-acting analgesics work by diffusing from the blood to the brain and spinal cord where they influence pain-conducting pathways. There is usually a strong relationship between the concentration of the drug in plasma and its effects in the central nervous system. For this reason the concentration of the drug in plasma is measured to provide an objective estimate of the likely effects of a drug regime.

Figure 13/3 shows the effects of irregularly given drugs on plasma

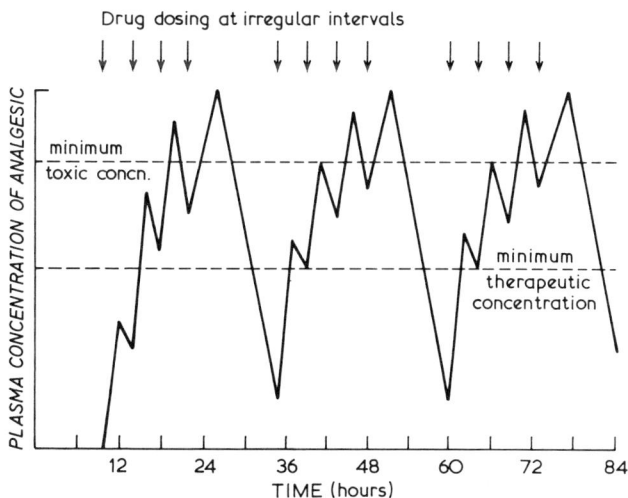

Fig. 13/3   Blood levels with irregular, or 'prn', doses of analgesics

concentrations. It can be seen that not only does the patient suffer long periods without effective analgesia, but that these may be interspersed by periods with increased side-effects. This is because putting periods of pain in between the periods of analgesia tends to lower the patient's threshold for pain, thereby increasing his demands for analgesia.

If, because of the patient's age or disease, the duration of an analgesic cannot be anticipated, then this type of patient-controlled, on-demand analgesic regime may be the safest to use, despite the shortcomings already expressed.

Volatile analgesia

The volatile analgesics trilene and methoxyflurane, as well as the gaseous analgesic mixture Entonox, would all be given *only* on patient demand. Even in quite modest doses, these agents are all capable of inducing anaesthesia in a proportion of patients.

Entonox is particularly rapid acting, yet even it takes 3 to 4 minutes to build up to an analgesic level in the patient. Agents such as this tend to be used for intermittently painful conditions, such as labour pains, or short, painful procedures, such as wound dressings and removal of drains.

CONTINUOUS ADMINISTRATION

Continuous infusions of drugs for analgesia may be given intravenously, intramuscularly, subcutaneously, epidurally or even spinally into the cerebrospinal fluid. The essential feature is a continuous flow of the drug to the patient, which allows continuous absorption into the blood rather than intermittently. This has the advantage that the patient cannot find the analgesia completely wearing off at any time. In other words, the patient can be kept pain-free continuously.

Plasma concentration

Figure 13/4 shows the changes in plasma concentrations of drugs given by continuous infusion, when the infusions are started, and when they are stopped. The line, representing plasma concentration after the infusion starts, also demonstrates what happens when the rate of infusion is increased. Initially there is a rapid change, which gets slower and slower, until it settles at the new, higher, level. The effect is both self-limiting and predictable. Similarly, when the infusion is discontinued, or slowed down, initially there is a rapid fall

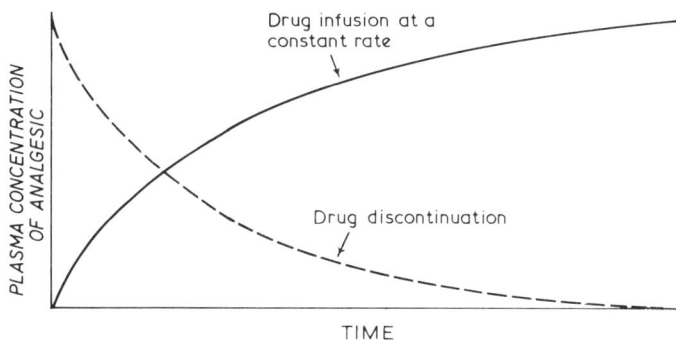

Fig. 13/4   The effects of starting or stopping an intravenous infusion of a drug

in the concentration, which slows down progressively until it reaches its new, lower, level. In practice, when an infusion of an analgesic such as fentanyl is started, it may take 2 to 3 hours before the plasma concentrations have stopped rising. If, during this time, the patient started to show unacceptable side-effects they would come on gradually and progressively, giving the nursing staff ample warning and time to adjust, or turn off, the infusion. The analgesic effects of the infusion wear off in a similarly progressive and predictable way. After 48 hours of a continuous infusion of fentanyl the analgesic effects usually wear off about 1 hour after stopping the infusion.

Infusion problems
Continuous infusions as described have three main problems. *First*, it is vitally important that the infusion rate is rigidly controlled otherwise an entire reservoir of drug prescribed to last several hours may be accidentally infused in a few minutes. Syringe pumps, infusion pumps and electrical drip controllers are all able to keep the infusion rate strictly controlled for long periods of time. They are, however, expensive. A less expensive way is to use a burette containing one hour's supply of the analgesic, which is allowed to infuse (intravenously) over 60 minutes, after which the ward nurse refills it with the supply for the next hour. The advantage here is that, should the burette accidentally infuse its entire contents over a few minutes, the dose of drug in the burette would be relatively small, and so would be most unlikely to cause serious problems.

The *second* problem of continuous infusion regimes is that they do not take account of variations in the patient's need for analgesic. There is no 'feedback' from the patient relating to the drug effectiveness. Patients on these regimes require careful observation, particularly during the first few hours, to ensure that the regime is appropriate for their needs. In our hospital, patients on continuous infusions are checked about 2 hours after starting one, with a view to adjusting the prescription to a higher or lower infusion rate. As the pain experienced by the patient gradually gets less so the rate of infusion may need to be reduced. If patients are given such continuous infusions for several days, the dose may need to be adjusted according to the incidence and severity of side-effects such as sedation or nausea, *rather* than the quality of pain relief.

The *third* problem is related to the slow and predictable onset of the drug's effects. With a fixed infusion, most drugs would level out after 2 to 4 hours, consequently the maximum effect of the regime would only be felt some 2 to 4 hours after starting the regime, while the patient's pain would probably be at its worst during this period. One of the criteria for the ideal postoperative analgesic regime is that it should rapidly achieve analgesia; it is obvious that the simple infusion described above does not do so.

Figure 13/5a illustrates the typical plasma levels of an analgesic when a simple infusion is started and run. Figure 13/5b shows what would happen if, in the same patient, the infusion was started at a much higher flow rate initially, and was then turned down to the maintenance rate. The high initial flow rate causes the plasma levels to rise much faster than with the simple infusion, so that the patient has analgesia provided more quickly. There are several methods available for deciding how fast the initial infusion should run, and for how long. The authors have found that the initial high infusion rate is best run at a speed related to the delay in the drug's onset time, and time to peak effect. The patient's report of pain relief (with the proviso that the respiratory rate should not be allowed to fall to a dangerously slow rate) is an excellent indicator for turning the high infusion rate down to the low basal rate.

For morphine given intravenously, the authors usually start the infusion at a rate of 0.5mg/minute; for pethidine, 5mg/minute; and for fentanyl, 10micrograms/minute. These dosages usually work well, and over the first 10 to 15 minutes after a major operation, a patient may obtain significant analgesia, allowing him to cough and breathe deeply, without pain (Fig. 13/6). This state is then maintained by the continuous infusion of a much lower maintenance dose

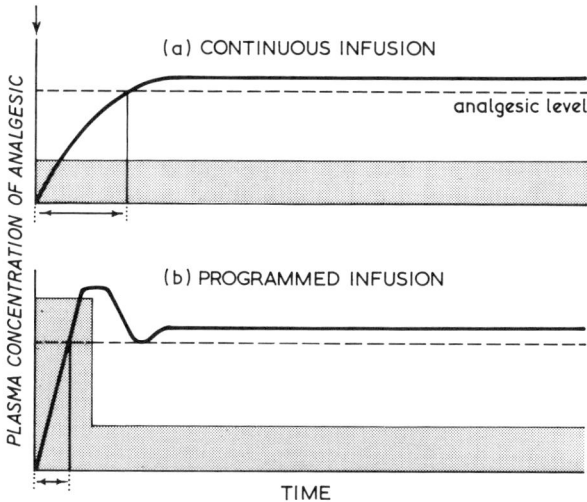

Fig. 13/5   Blood levels with intravenous infusion of narcotic
analgesics. The double-ended arrow indicates the delay before
analgesia is achieved. The shaded area represents the rate of
infusion

(usually one-tenth of the high rate) for as long as is necessary, which
often coincides with the time when the patient starts to move out of
bed (Fig. 13/7). One of the functions of good postoperative analgesia
is to allow a patient to be up and about as quickly as possible; if,
therefore, the patient is ready to be mobile, but still has a constant
analgesic infusion which severely limits him, it is better to sacrifice
the infusion than to hold back his mobilisation.

COMBINATION OF REPEATED DOSES AND
CONTINUOUS ADMINISTRATION

Patient controlled syringe pumps
Small bedside microcomputers are now available which can control
the rate and depth of infusion of analgesic to the individual patient.
In the United Kingdom the simplest device available is the Cardiff
Palliator (Fig. 13/8). By pressing a large button twice in one second,
the device delivers small incremental doses of the analgesic to the
patient when he requires pain relief. Of the more complex machines

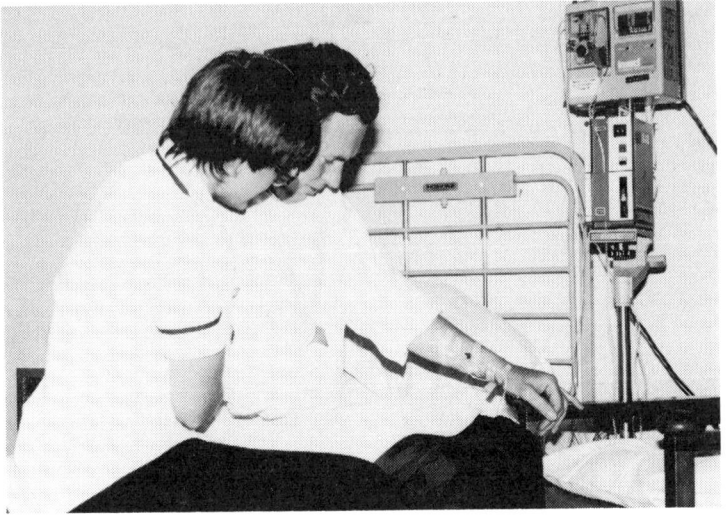

Fig. 13/6   A continuous infusion of narcotic analgesic allows this patient to cough and breathe deeply without pain on the morning following surgery

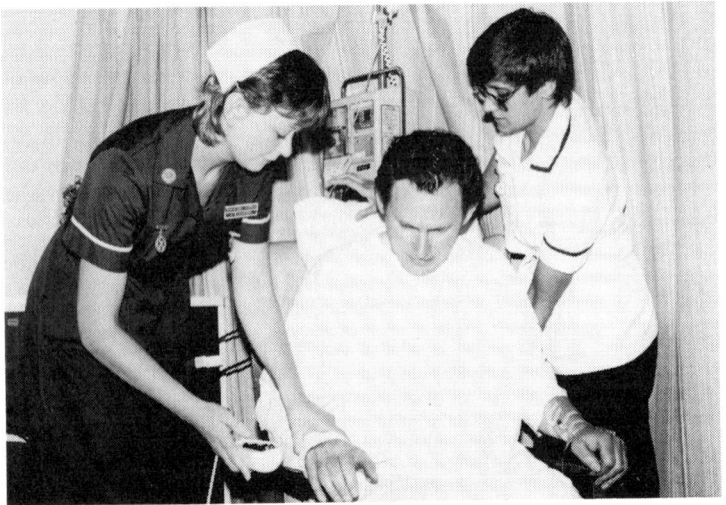

Fig. 13/7   Early mobilisation from bed to chair is achieved with minimum discomfort

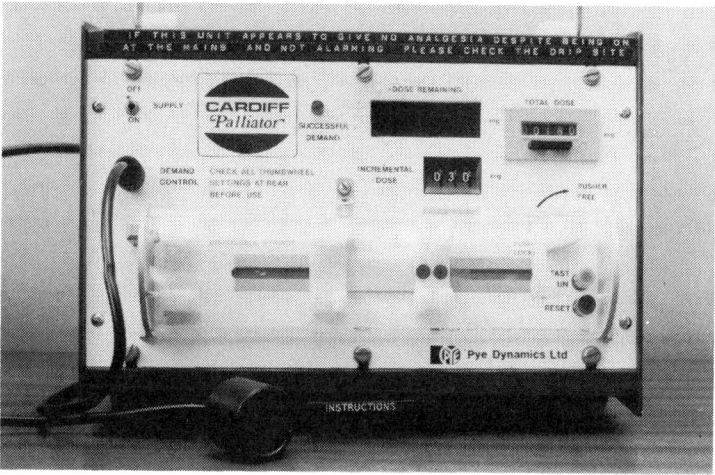

Fig. 13/8 The Cardiff
Palliator

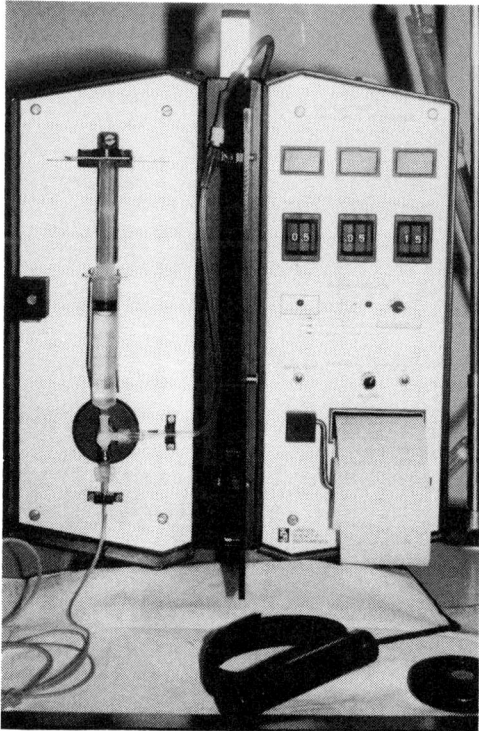

Fig. 13/9 The On
Demand Analgesic
Computer (ODAC)

available, the Janssen Scientific Instruments' On Demand Analgesic Computer (ODAC) (Fig. 13/9) may give a continuous background infusion as well as the demanded doses.

Finally, there is a third level of sophistication which can tailor the background infusion to the level of the patient's apparent needs. This is done by allowing each patient to demand small intravenous doses of the analgesic at intervals, and, depending upon the rate of his demand, the computer increases, or decreases, the rate of a background infusion of the drug. In this way the number of demands for additional analgesia may be minimised while making provision for the analgesic infusion to turn itself down slowly when it is no longer required.

Chapter Fourteen

ROUTES OF ADMINISTRATION
FOR ANALGESICS

To achieve effective analgesia using drugs, it is necessary to administer the chosen drug by the most appropriate route. Side-effects which result from the administration of medication will be those due to the technique used to administer the drug, together with any problems which may be encountered with the particular drug. The chosen route of administration should be the least invasive one which will deliver the drug of choice reliably to the patient using the chosen regime. The least invasive route which is most used is the oral one, for both tablets and syrups.

NON-INVASIVE ROUTES

Oral

Following major surgery, and particularly bowel surgery, patients often develop an ileus. While the bowel is non-active, anything which is ingested into the stomach is unlikely to be propelled into the small bowel where most absorption takes place. For this reason, delivering medicines by the oral route during this early phase after major surgery tends to be futile and possibly dangerous. The medication may build up in the stomach until the ileus stops, then a large depot of unabsorbed drug may suddenly be propelled into the small bowel, to be absorbed all at once. For this reason, oral pain-killers are only given to patients immediately following minor surgery, or several days after major surgery when any postoperative ileus has worn off.

The administration of syrups and other liquids seldom presents problems, but, there may be some with patients taking tablets and capsules. If capsules and tablets are administered to patients who are lying flat, a high proportion may stick in the lower portion of the oesophagus, where they dissolve, causing an oesophagitis, and are poorly absorbed. Similarly, giving patients less than 100ml of water with their tablets and capsules, also leads to a high incidence of their not getting into the stomach before dissolving. From this it is clear that for reliable absorption of oral medication, it should be given with about 100ml of water to the patient in a sitting or upright position.

The oral route of administration usually works relatively slowly and so is inappropriate for patients in severe acute pain, who require rapid analgesia. Many drugs are metabolised into inactive compounds in the gut walls and in the liver before the active drug can get into the systemic circulation. This is why most analgesics are less active when given orally, compared with the same drug given by injection. The oral dose of these drugs is therefore higher than the comparable parenteral dose. All the narcotics show this effect.

Sublingual
The sublingual route requires medication to be left under the tongue until absorbed. Once absorbed into the mucosa of the tongue, the drug may either be released into the circulation immediately, or there may be a delay before it appears in the blood.

Glyceryl trinitrate tablets are prescribed sublingually for angina, and may start to work within a few minutes of putting them under the tongue.

Buprenorphine is a potent narcotic analgesic given by the sublingual route, which does not start to work for over an hour after administration. Buprenorphine tablets take about 10 minutes to dissolve under the tongue and during this time the drug is absorbed into the mucosa. It then appears to stay there for a long time before being released into the circulation. While sublingual buprenorphine would be inappropriate for someone in severe acute pain in need of immediate relief, the route works well for maintenance of analgesia, after the first dose is given parenterally to obtain a rapid onset of action.

Buprenorphine is an example of a drug which is metabolised in the gut wall and liver when given orally; to be effective, therefore, the oral dose must be large. If the sublingual tablets are, by error, given orally, or accidentally swallowed, they will appear to have little or no effect on the patient's pain. This is an example of a drug being given by the wrong route, with unexpected results.

Inhalation

Entonox and trilene are both administered by inhalation via demand-only systems which means that both will only be delivered to a mask if an air-tight seal is maintained between the mask and the patient's face, and the patient actively inspires from the mask. Both require a mask which should be held in place by the patient himself, because both agents are capable of anaesthetising if given for too long. Provided the mask is held by the patient without assistance, it will fall away from his face when he becomes drowsy, and the agent will no longer be delivered. Inhalational agents of this kind should only be given by personnel trained in their use, as patients may easily be under- or overdosed if not supervised correctly (Fig. 14/1).

The advantages of the inhalational route include its rapid onset of action and the fact that the analgesic drug can be excreted, without metabolism, from the lungs. This means that the effects can wear off

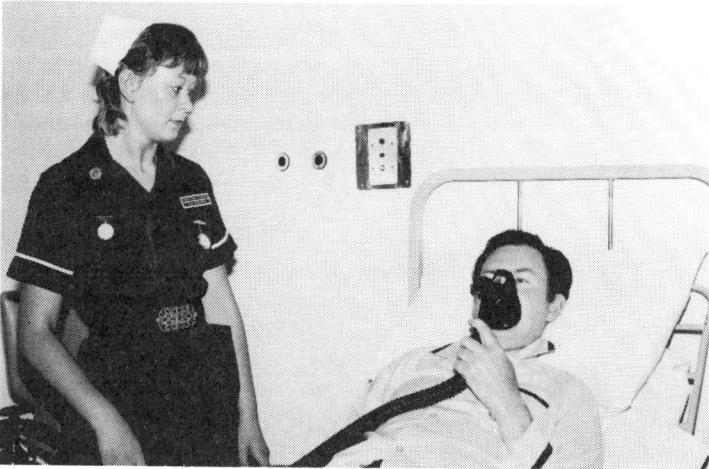

Fig. 14/1   Delivering Entonox. Entonox is delivered by demand: the agent is delivered to the mask when an air-tight seal is maintained between the patient's face and the mask. The mask should only be held in place by the patient and inhalational agents should be supervised by personnel trained in their use

predictably in a relatively short period of time. Entonox is widely used in obstetrics and in ambulances, because it provides analgesia of rapid onset and short duration while also giving 50 per cent oxygen. It is also used on wards for relatively short, painful procedures, e.g. wound dressings.

The disadvantages to this route of drug administration include the need for special equipment as well as trained personnel to supervise the giving of drugs by it (Fig. 14/2). Another disadvantage is that the exhaled analgesic is difficult to remove from the ward atmosphere leading to a noticeable smell and a pollution hazard. Current legislation recommends that anti-pollution systems be used wherever possible when agents of this kind are used. This is both impractical and expensive on the postoperative ward. Long-term continuous use of both Entonox and trilene over a period of days may be associated with serious side-effects, such as bone marrow depression and liver failure, for the patients. These agents, and hence this route, should be used only for short periods of time.

Rectal
The rectal mucosa is well able to absorb lipid-soluble drugs, yet this route has remained unpopular in the United Kingdom, despite its

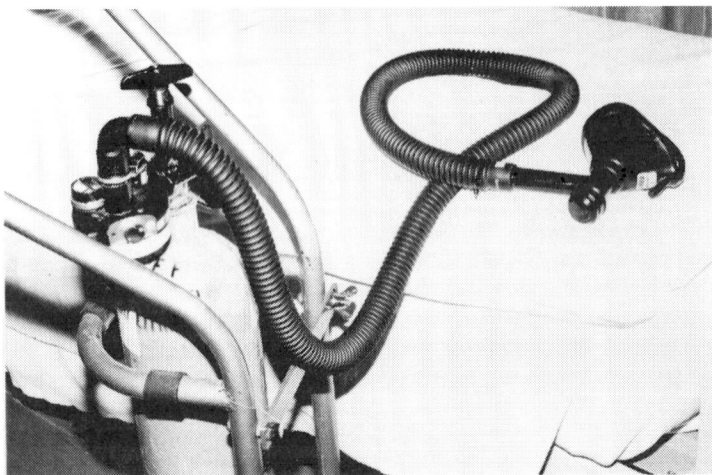

Fig. 14/2   Entonox equipment which may be used on wards for short, painful procedures

widespread use on the Continent. Because of its unpopularity, there are few analgesic preparations available for use in this way.

Non-steroidal anti-inflammatory drugs, which can cause problems with gastric bleeding when given orally, may be given as rectal suppositories instead, with fewer side-effects.

Patients in pain who are unable to take oral medication, because of vomiting, or because their original pathology, or surgery prevents oral medication from being absorbed properly may be effectively treated with rectal analgesics. In general, rectal analgesics are used for patients with chronic or terminal pain, who require analgesia which is long lasting, but without recourse to injections. In such patients the advantages of this route obviously outweigh social prejudices.

INVASIVE ROUTES

Intramuscular and subcutaneous injections
These two routes are by far the most commonly used for giving analgesics to postoperative patients. They have the advantage of requiring only minimal technical skill to carry out the injections, and are relatively reliable methods of delivering depots of analgesics to patients who are not able to tolerate oral medication. Giving an injection is not without risk, and the deeper the injection the less control the administrator has over precisely where it goes. Intramuscular injections may cause problems if the needle pierces underlying structures, such as blood vessels and nerves. Nerves may be physically damaged by the needle, or be irritated by having the analgesic injected into, or on to, them. Major nerve damage is rare but minor degrees of nerve damage may lead to long-lasting neuritis, with consequent pain and loss of sensation in the affected distribution of the nerve. Nurses are taught the optimum areas into which intramuscular injections may be administered without damage. For example, injection into the upper outer quadrant of the buttock reduces the likelihood of damage to the sciatic nerve.

Simple piercing of a blood vessel may result in leakage of blood into the surrounding tissues causing a haematoma. This will probably be worse if an artery, rather than a vein, is punctured. In both cases, the patient will have a painful swelling. Haematoma may be a serious problem in patients with clotting disorders, or those on anticoagulant therapy.

Another problem associated with vascular penetration is that of intravascular injection. However, if the syringe is adequately aspirated before injection of its contents this is unlikely. Intravenous injection of a dose of analgesic, meant to be given as an intramuscular depot, lasting several hours, may cause the sudden onset of respiratory depression and sedation far in excess of that expected. Intra-arterial injection of the analgesic may initially cause quite different problems. Small and medium sized arteries have very active smooth muscle in their walls, which may contract violently in response to intra-arterial injections of almost anything other than bland isotonic electrolyte solutions. This arterial spasm may be quite painful in itself and may be made more painful by the development of ischaemic changes distal to the site of injection, where blood flow from the artery has become reduced because of the spasm. Puncturing arterial walls, sending them into spasm, and injecting drugs into the arteries may all cause damage to the inner lining layer of the artery. The clotting mechanisms of the body are designed to recognise damage of this kind as a possible source of haemorrhage and so will start to form a blood clot at the site of the damage. The sudden reduction in blood flow may cause permanent and serious damage to those tissues normally supplied by the artery.

The ideal site of an intramuscular injection should be a substantial area of muscle with a good blood supply, but which has no major nerves, arteries or veins running under that portion to be injected. This allows the injected drug to diffuse into the muscle itself and be absorbed into the bloodstream.

Both the subcutaneous and intramuscular routes may have a reduced uptake into the blood of patients who are in hypovolaemic shock due to undertransfusion after major surgery, or who are cold after a long operation during which measures to keep the patient warm were not used. In all these instances blood flow will be shunted away from the skin and muscles, towards the vital organs. If injections of powerful analgesics are given, but not absorbed, they may be stored in the tissues, until the blood flow to those tissues is restored. By this time, more injections of the powerful analgesics may have been given, leading to quite a large depot of the drug suddenly being absorbed as blood volume is restored, or when the patient warms up. In these circumstances, where absorption may be impaired from skin and muscles, these routes are probably not the most appropriate to use.

Intravenous injection

In the United Kingdom only specially trained nurses are allowed to give drugs intravenously. This is for several reasons:

1. The technical problems of injecting into a vein.
2. The problems associated with injection into the wrong place. There is always the possibility of mistaking an artery for a vein and injecting the drug accidentally into the artery, causing all the problems discussed under this heading in the previous section.
3. The problem of speed of onset of the drug's actions when given intravenously. One of the major advantages of giving analgesics intravenously is that they start to work within minutes of the injection. Paradoxically it also means that if they are given too suddenly, the patient may suddenly start to exhibit major side-effects, such as respiratory depression, before staff are aware of what is happening.

The intravenous route has the advantage of predictability, in that it does not rely on the gradual absorption of a depot of drug from the bowel or an area of muscle (Fig. 14/3). When an analgesic is given intravenously, it goes directly into the blood with no intervening stages. If a correctly given dose of drug is considered too large for a patient, then simply not giving any more causes an immediate decrease in the amount of drug in the patient's blood. Shock, cold and hypovolaemia should not alter the predictability of analgesics given this way.

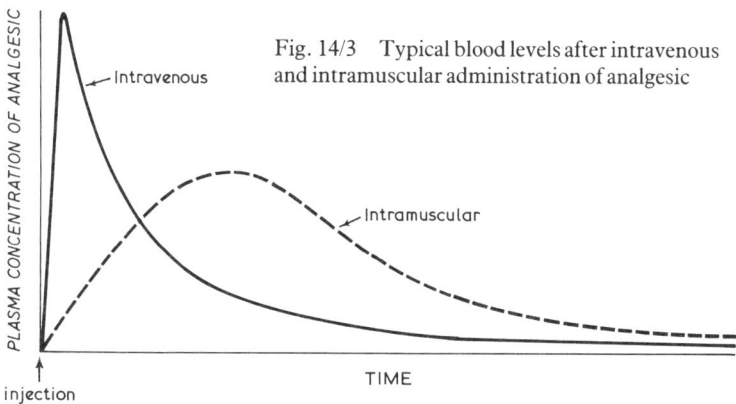

Fig. 14/3   Typical blood levels after intravenous and intramuscular administration of analgesic

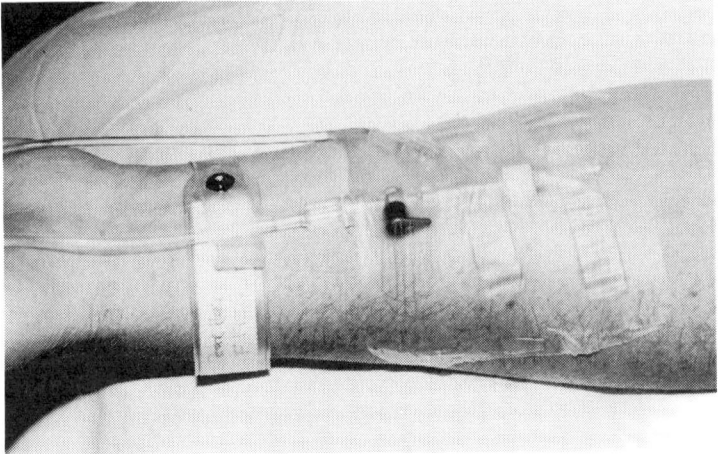

Fig. 14/4   Analgesia via continuous intravenous infusion. A Y-connection is attached to the intravenous line. The analgesic enters the connection and is prevented from passing up the intravenous line by the one-way valve

The authors have found the intravenous route to be one of the best for providing rapid, effective analgesia after surgery, which can then be continued over the postoperative period by a continuous infusion of the same analgesic, also delivered intravenously (Fig. 14/4). The advantages and disadvantages of these regimes are discussed in Chapter 13.

Epidural
Figure 14/5 shows the epidural space which is within the bony spine, but outside the dura which covers the spinal cord and keeps in the cerebrospinal fluid. Local anaesthetics and narcotic analgesics may be administered into the epidural space of a patient through a fine plastic catheter inserted under sterile conditions. This procedure can be used for women in labour, patients with chronic back pain, and patients who are going to suffer severe postoperative pain. Using a special technique, the sterile plastic catheter is inserted through a ligament-covered foramen in the bony spine until its tip lies just outside the dura. The proximal portion of the catheter is taped to the patient's skin, so that the relevant drug may be administered through the catheter and then into the epidural space.

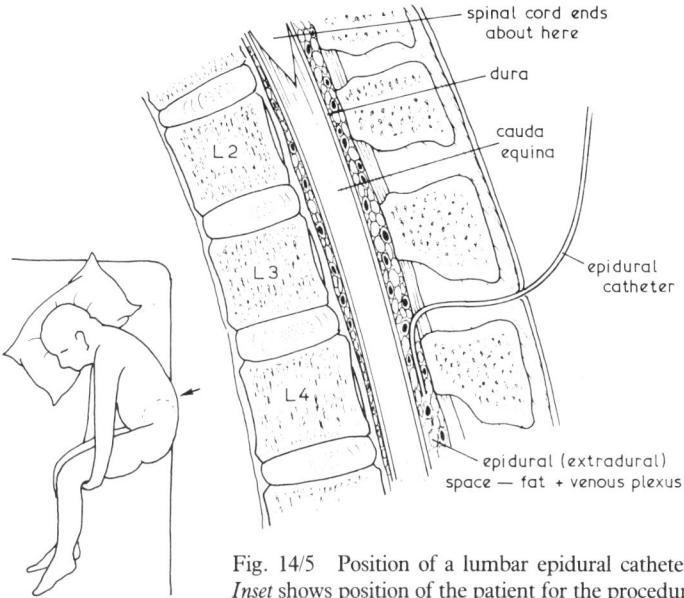

Fig. 14/5   Position of a lumbar epidural catheter. *Inset* shows position of the patient for the procedure

The epidural space is used because it allows drugs to be injected near to the spinal cord and the nerves around it. The drug then diffuses across the dura, through the cerebrospinal fluid, and into the spinal cord or its associated nerves. This is achieved without puncturing the dura thus ensuring no leakage of the cerebrospinal fluid or introduction of infection into it. Local anaesthetics administered in this way freeze the afferent and efferent nerves in the region of the epidural catheter, which may result in loss of sensation and control of the muscles supplied.

For women in labour, an epidural catheter may be inserted into the low lumbar region so that the local anaesthetic will freeze the nerves coming from the uterus and vagina. This allows labour and subsequent delivery to be pain-free. It may also numb the legs as they are supplied by the same nerve roots.

An epidural catheter may be inserted into the thoracic region for patients undergoing thoracic or upper abdominal surgery. Either a local anaesthetic or narcotic analgesic may be administered through the catheter to provide pain relief. Local anaesthetics will block conduction of nerve impulses, while the narcotics interfere only with the passage of pain impulses, leaving other sensations and motor power normal. The quality of analgesia with narcotics is very good, but slightly less than that with the local anaesthetics. Surgery may be performed under a local anaesthetic epidural, whereas it would be impossible with a narcotic one.

Nurses have to be specially trained, and then 'licensed' or certificated to administer the prescribed drug down the previously placed catheter. The nurse may *not* insert the catheter.

Scrupulous aseptic technique *must* be used; the introduction of any infected material into the catheter could result in the formation of an epidural abscess and severe neurological damage to the patient. The skin at the site of the catheter insertion must be regularly checked for early signs of redness and infection.

Before any injection of a drug the catheter should always be checked visually for the presence of blood which, if seen, would suggest that the catheter tip may have penetrated a blood vessel. This may happen at any time and not simply when the catheter is placed in the epidural space. If an epidural catheter is seen to have blood in it, drugs should never be injected as the entire dose may go intravenously, possibly causing a life-threatening reaction. Alternatively, the drug may enter an epidural artery, possibly causing it to thrombose or go into spasm leading to neurological problems.

Occasionally, the epidural catheter erodes through the dura, allowing the tip to lie in the cerebrospinal fluid. When this has happened, there may be a tell-tale length of clear fluid within the catheter, or some may be easily aspirated into it using an empty syringe before giving the top-up dose. If this situation arises, any dose of local anaesthetic going into this space would spread further than if the same dose were to go into the epidural space. A typical epidural top-up would be 10ml. This might spread some five or six spinal segments above and below the site of the catheter. If 10ml is injected into the cerebrospinal solution it could spread to affect the whole length of the spinal cord. Should a local anaesthetic be injected in this way, total body paralysis, including inability to breathe, would begin within minutes of the injection. The sympathetic nerves, because they have the finest diameter, are most readily affected by local anaesthetics and under the above circumstances would be the first nerves to lose their function, leading to a rapid, massive fall in blood pressure within minutes of the spinal injection.

From these comments it is quite obvious that epidural top-up injections require precision and care. However, they do have many advantages in terms of providing high quality analgesia to patients with the most severe pain. Despite the serious hazards mentioned they *do* have a good safety record because of the high standards of care and delivery which are insisted upon.

Chapter Fifteen

UNDERSTANDING THE MISUSE OF DRUGS ACT 1971

Many of the powerful analgesics used for the relief of severe pain are termed Controlled Drugs. There are special regulations which limit their supply, control their storage, and govern their prescription and administration. Nurses who use these drugs have to comply with an Act of Parliament which few of them will ever have seen. The Act and its amendments are long, and cover many drugs, most of which are not used for pain management. The authors have tried to summarise the main features of the Act and its amendments as they apply to the management of patients with acute pain.

These regulations apply particularly to Controlled Drugs when used in the *community*. They do, however, act as strong recommendations for the use of such drugs in hospitals. In 1958 a report, *Control of Controlled Drugs and Poisons in Hospitals* (the Aitken Report), made a list of recommendations concerning the administration of all drugs in hospitals. This report was followed by a number of circulars and reports (see p. 145).

The majority of these reports are advisory, and their recommendations have been put into practice by local health authorities and at individual hospitals in the United Kingdom. There are many local variations in hospital practices concerning the control of medicines in general and Controlled Drugs in particular. These local regulations are concerned mainly with the safeguarding of members of staff, such as the ward sister or 'nurse in charge of the ward', who will be responsible legally for possessing the Controlled Drugs. Variations in practice may exist within the same hospital depending on local requirements. For instance, there may be quite different requirements between the wards and the operating theatre for witnessing and recording the administration of Controlled Drugs. Failure to comply with these local requirements which are not covered by the Misuse of Drugs Act may result in disciplinary hearings.

The Misuse of Drugs Act 1971 came into operation on 1st July 1973, and was designed to consolidate and extend previous legislation as well as control the export, import, production, supply and possession of dangerous or otherwise harmful drugs. The Act was also designed to deal with the control and treatment of addicts, and to promote education and research relating to drug dependence.

There are four schedules of drugs covered by the Act, but only *Schedule 2* drugs are Controlled Drugs. The term Controlled Drug refers to any drug or substance listed in that Schedule. The Schedule is divided into three classes (Class A, Class B and Class C) on the basis of their decreasing order of harmfulness. This division into classes is done to simplify the penalties incurred by anyone committing an offence under the Act.

Schedule 1 (which excludes preparations for injection) includes certain preparations of Controlled Drugs such as morphine, codeine and pholcodeine, which are combined in such small amounts with other substances so as to make their abuse-potential negligible, and their extraction from the preparation very difficult. These preparations have no restrictions laid on them regarding their sale, import, export, possession or administration. No prescription is needed to obtain them and no record need be kept of their supply or administration. A typical example is Kaolin and Morphine Mixture BP.

Schedule 2 drugs include the opiates, such as heroin, morphine and methadone, and the major stimulants such as the amphetamines. A special licence is needed to import or export these drugs. A pharmacist may supply these drugs to a patient only on the authority of a prescription written in the correct manner and issued by a registered medical practitioner. These drugs may only be administered to patients by a registered medical practitioner or dentist, or by a person acting in accordance with the directions of a registered medical practitioner or dentist. There are strict requirements concerning the safe custody of these drugs in pharmacies and on wards, and the regulations also cover the way in which these drugs may be disposed of or destroyed. Controlled Drugs must be kept in specially marked containers and a strict record kept of their supply and administration.

Schedule 3 drugs include a small number of minor stimulant drugs such as benzphetamine, as well as other drugs which are not thought likely to be so harmful when misused as the drugs in Schedules 2 and 4. The controls which apply to Schedule 2 also apply to Schedule 3 drugs, except that there is a difference in the classes of people who are allowed to possess and supply them; the requirements concerning their destruction do not apply; no records need be kept in the register of Controlled Drugs; and they may be manufactured by registered people.

Schedule 4 drugs include the hallucinogenic drugs such as LSD and cannabis, and are not relevant to this book.

REQUISITIONS FOR CONTROLLED DRUGS

Only the sister, or acting sister, in charge of the ward, operating theatre, or other department of a hospital, can requisition Controlled Drugs from the pharmacy. The requisition *must* fulfil the following:

be in writing
be signed by the sister
specify the total amount of the drug required.

The ward sister must retain a copy or a note of the requisition for two years, and have it available for inspection should that be necessary. The person who dispenses and supplies the drug must mark the requisition to show that it has been complied with, and must then retain that record for two years also.

In the case of a nursing home the matron, or acting matron, must have her requisition countersigned by a registered medical practitioner or dentist working at that nursing home.

There are occasions when the person requesting the Controlled Drugs cannot himself collect the drugs from the supplier or pharmacy. In these cases an 'authorised person' should be sent, or a statement in writing, signed by the person who made the requisition to the effect that the person carrying the statement is empowered by the signatory to the requisition to receive the drug on his behalf.

The term 'authorised person' is vague, and hospitals have interpreted this in different ways.

SAFE CUSTODY OF CONTROLLED DRUGS

Any person having possession of a Controlled Drug to which the safe custody regulations apply, namely Schedules 2, 3, and 4, must ensure that it is kept in a locked receptacle which can be opened only by himself or a person authorised by him.

On the ward this means that Controlled Drugs must be stored in a separate cupboard which has its own key. In practice, most hospital regulations stipulate that the Controlled Drugs cupboard is itself locked within a cupboard for internal medicines.

Only the sister, or charge nurse, in charge of the ward is legally entitled to possess the Controlled Drugs there, and hence to hold the keys to the Controlled Drugs cupboard. However, the regulations allow for a suitable nominee to hold the keys in the absence, away from the ward, of these persons. The definition of a suitable nominee is vague and wide variations will be found.

REGISTERS AND RECORDS OF CONTROLLED DRUGS

An entry in a register of Controlled Drugs must be made for each quantity of a Schedule 2 or Schedule 4 drug which is obtained or supplied whether for administration or otherwise. Entries must be in chronological order, in a bound book which is kept always on the premises. No alterations, crossing out or cancellations of any kind may be made, other than by notes in the margins or at the foot of the page. Every entry must be in indelible ink and must be dated. A running record of stocks held should also be kept, even if not legally required.

All registers of Controlled Drugs must be kept for at least two years after the last entry.

PRESCRIPTIONS FOR CONTROLLED DRUGS

A *prescription* means the prescription written by a registered medical practitioner or dentist for the medical treatment of a single individual. No prescription is required for Schedule 1 drugs.

A prescription for Schedule 2 and Schedule 3 drugs must not be issued unless it fulfils the following requirements:

1. It is in ink or be otherwise indelible. It must be written and signed by the doctor or dentist issuing it, and be dated by him.

2. It is labelled 'for dental treatment only' if issued by a dentist.
3. It has (written on it in the handwriting of the prescriber) the name and address of the person for whose treatment it is issued, unless the person is a patient in a hospital or nursing home when the prescription is written on the bed card or case sheet.
4. It specifies the dose to be taken and, either the total quantity of the drug to be supplied (in words *and* figures), or the number of dosage units (in words *and* figures), as appropriate. In the case of preparations of Controlled Drugs, the prescription must state the form and, where appropriate, the strength of the preparation.
5. It specifies the amount of each instalment and the intervals between each instalment, if a Controlled Drug is prescribed as a total quantity to be given in instalments.

A Controlled Drug must not be supplied before the date specified on the prescription, and it should not be supplied later than 13 weeks after the date specified by the prescription. The date at the time of dispensing must be marked on a prescription for a Controlled Drug.

Most hospitals now have a standardised system for the checking, recording and administering of all drugs to in-patients. Most hospitals use a system requiring the administration to be performed by one nurse and witnessed and recorded by a second nurse or doctor. Similarly, most hospitals require the administration of a Controlled Drug by a nurse to be witnessed and recorded by a second nurse. There are local variations as to the grade of staff who are allowed to act as a witness or administrator in these procedures. Operating theatre areas may have quite different local regulations concerning the witnessing of Controlled Drug administration, because of the difficulties created by anaesthetic practice.

MIDWIVES AND THE USE OF PETHIDINE

A certified midwife, as defined in the Midwives Act 1951 and subsequently amended (England 1973; and Scotland 1972), who has notified the local supervising authority of her intention to practise may, as far as is necessary for the practice of her profession or employment as a midwife, possess and administer pethidine.

Supplies may be made only to her, or possessed by her, on the authority of a 'midwife's supply order' which is an order in writing specifying the name and occupation of the midwife obtaining the pethidine, the purpose for which it is required, and the total quantity to be supplied. It must be signed by a doctor who is either authorised in writing by the local supervising authority for the purposes of this particular regulation, or by a person appointed under the Midwives Act 1951 to exercise supervision over certified midwives in that area.

Whenever a midwife obtains a supply of pethidine, she must enter in a book kept by her solely for this purpose the date, name and address of the supplier from whom it was obtained, and the form in which it was obtained. When she administers pethidine to a patient she must record in the same book, as soon as is practicable, the name and address of the patient, the amount administered and the form in which it was administered.

When the midwife is working in a hospital ward, she should follow the code of practice used on those wards concerning the possession and administration of Controlled Drugs such as pethidine.

RELEVANT CIRCULARS

DHSS (1970). *Measures for Controlling Drugs in the Wards* (Annis Gillie Report), HM(70)36. HMSO, London.

HC(77)16, *Amendments to Misuse of Drugs Regulations* (1973). HMSO, London.

The Labelling Regulations, SI 1762, HN(76)205 (1976). HMSO, London.

Ministry of Health (1958). *Control of Controlled Drugs and Poisons in Hospital* (Aitken Report). HMSO, London.

Misuse of Drugs Regulations, SI No 796.(1973). HMSO, London.

Security of Drugs Liable to Misuse, HM(70)1.

Chapter Sixteen

ACHIEVING ANALGESIA WITHOUT DRUGS

THE PLACEBO RESPONSE

A placebo is a 'false' or dummy treatment which may be given in place of a therapy which is expected, or is known, to work. A placebo treatment may be in any form, for example a tablet containing inactive chalk powder, or a therapeutic talk with a patient which deliberately misses out certain key topics. A placebo response is that which occurs when a patient appears to have had a successful treatment, although, unknown to him, the active part was missing. Placebos given for pain result in positive responses in approximately one-third of instances, despite the fact that no active analgesic was given.

Clearly if no active treatment is given then the side-effects are likely to be few and for this reason placebo analgesia is used clinically. Chapter 3 described how the response to pain may be mediated by the descending inhibitory pathways in the spinal cord. The analgesia produced by the placebo response may be reversed by giving naloxone. This suggests that the placebo response to pain is related to the release of naturally occurring opiates.

As there is no effective way of picking out the placebo responders in advance, the use of placebos alone is of limited value. If a group of patients in pain were given nothing but placebos, about 60 per cent of them would remain in pain which would be entirely unethical. However, placebo analgesia can be used effectively *in addition* to active treatment for postoperative pain. In general, placebo analgesia can be provided by all members of staff who are looking after patients through their being cheerful, informative, optimistic and enthusiastic about treatment prescribed.

DISTRACTION

Awareness of pain may be decreased by drawing attention away from it. Distracting patients with conversation or by involving them in concentration on a pleasant experience will help to make the patient less sensitive to pain. Distraction is frequently available for patients being cared for in a busy ward where there is constant activity. Patients nursed away from others, in single rooms, may be more aware of their discomfort for this reason. Just as attention can be drawn away from unpleasant experiences of pain, so too can it be focused on to how much pain is being felt. If someone discusses the amount of discomfort a patient is likely to feel when a painful procedure is being performed he is likely to be more sensitive to it. Most mothers learn the art of distraction when coping with hurt or frustrated young children and use it to advantage. Those caring for patients in pain will find that distraction often assists in providing significant analgesia.

RELAXATION

Much of the pain experienced after surgery is generated by the incision through the skin and muscle. Any tension in the affected muscles will give rise to pain. Therefore, teaching the patient to relax and showing him methods of movement which minimise the tension in wounded muscles may markedly reduce his pain after surgery. These techniques are usually taught by a physiotherapist but in many units the physiotherapist will also demonstrate how the nurse can contribute in this teaching.

METHODS REQUIRING EQUIPMENT OF SOME KIND

Counter-irritation

Most of us have at some time or other, tried to relieve a pain by rubbing the affected part, or by putting something warm or cold on it. Going to bed with a hot water bottle is a common remedy for dysmenorrhoea, which is widely practised because it appears to work, yet is rarely used in hospitals. These simple methods may work by distracting the patient's attention away from the pain, so reducing sensitivity to it. They may also work by stimulating the large sensory fibres from the affected part, which may then send their impulses to the dorsal horn of the spinal cord, to close the pain-gates (see Chapter 3).

Transcutaneous nerve stimulation (TNS)

The large sensory fibres may also be stimulated electrically through the skin, using small battery-powered stimulators which send their impulses through pairs of electrodes which are taped on to the skin, near the affected part, or near to those parts of the back to where the nerves will run. The large fibres have a lower electrical threshold for excitation and so can be stimulated electrically in this way, without stimulating the smaller diameter fibres which are usually associated with the conduction of painful impulses. Large fibre sensory input of this kind appears to close the spinal cord pain-gates and so reduces the painful sensation. Transcutaneous nerve stimulation (TNS) is widely used in the management of chronic pain conditions, and several trials have shown that it is of some benefit for patients with acute pain, such as postoperative pain, or labour pain (Fig. 16/1).

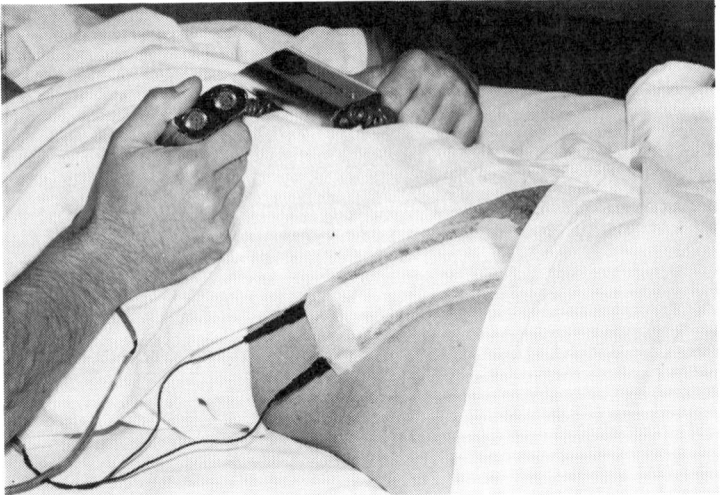

Fig. 16/1   Transcutaneous nerve stimulation. A patient operating the stimulator

Cryotherapy

Local anaesthetics have already been described as a method of reversibly stopping painful sensations from travelling along the sensory nerves to the central nervous system, to be perceived as pain. Nerve conduction may also be blocked by freezing the nerves. In much the same way that local anaesthetics affect small, pain-conducting nerves before they affect the larger nerves conducting other forms of sensation and motor impulses, so also does freezing preferentially affect these same small pain-conducting nerve fibres.

Simply cooling the affected part of the body, with ice packs or a freezing spray, may temporarily stop the nerves from functioning until the part warms up and the nerves regain their normal conductive properties. This effect is widely used in casualty departments and on the games field to stop minor bruises and sprains from hurting but its cooling effect is only temporary. If, however, the nerves are cooled until they freeze solid, then the frozen sections of nerve will die. If these sections are relatively short, they will regrow over a period of weeks or months, depending on the lengths of nerve frozen in the first place. This technique of cooling nerves until they freeze can be used during an operation such as thoracotomy, where the nerves involved in postoperative pain are relatively exposed and easy to reach. Alternatively, a freezing probe can be introduced under local anaesthetic to the site of the nerves involved in the pain. Cryotherapy of this kind may cause relatively long-lasting analgesia in a region for up to several months.

Acupuncture

Acupuncture may work either by distraction, or by stimulation of large sensory nerve fibres, which close the pain-gates in the spinal cord. Like TNS, acupuncture is quite widely practised for treating chronic painful conditions, but it is much less widely used in the United Kingdom for acute pain treatment.

Chapter Seventeen

RESEARCH INTO PAIN CONTROL

In 1976 a journalist wrote of his experiences following surgery and stated that the treatment of postoperative pain was 'the grave defect in English public hospital treatment . . . a cruel and callous disgrace'.

This account stimulated letters, editorials and review articles in the medical literature, nearly all of which stressed the inadequacy of postoperative pain-relief.

Research is undertaken because the investigator feels that there is a need to look closely at a subject to discover more about it. Research, or critical investigation, may involve scrutiny and review, exhaustive enquiry and cross-examination. It may also involve experimentation and trial.

Previously, *acute* pain has not received the same attention as chronic and terminal pain. This may be because both those who suffered acute pain, and those who relieved it, had rationalised the treatment. Acute pain tends to be short-lived (so perhaps doesn't matter so much), and many patients don't want to appear ungracious and so make no fuss. Surgeons are perhaps more concerned with the technical aspects of surgery, relegating responsibility for pain to junior doctors, who are inexperienced, and nurses, who are unable to prescribe. Both these groups may be complacent about pain after surgery, accepting it as inevitable, and, too often, withholding drugs when they should be given. Research in recent years has highlighted many of these areas of concern and given doctors and nurses the impetus to enquire into the problems of adequately controlling pain and to search for better ways of doing so.

Research into pain-relief is always directed at the sufferer, and has one ultimate goal – to improve on existing treatments. In this context the research has involved enquiry and questioning, not only of pain-relieving drugs and methods of administering them, but also of psychological influences affecting patients and those who care for them.

While some research aimed at pain-relief involves pain mechanisms and will be carried out in the laboratory by scientists, much of the knowledge gained in recent years and the subsequent understanding and treatment of acute pain has been undertaken with patients. It is, after all, the patient who knows what his pain is, and only the patient who can gauge the success of pain-relieving methods. In the past decade research into better control and management of pain after surgery has enabled newer methods of pain-relief to become publicised and put into practice by both doctors and nurses.

Research with patients in acute pain has to involve nurses. The nurse's role in such research may be one of three areas: she may just be there, aware that research is being carried out but not actively part of it; she may be actively involved, perhaps by taking requested observations or administering specific regimes; or she might herself be doing the research.

AWARENESS OF RESEARCH

Any patient who takes part in research must give his informed consent to do so. This means that the nature and purpose of the study, trial or experiment must be explained to the patient by the researcher or assistant. The researcher must be absolutely certain that the patient understands what is involved. If there is any reluctance on the part of the patient or his family, then pressure should not be put upon them as this would be both unethical and unfair.

When the research involves the patient in simply answering questions, the nature of the questions to be asked should be outlined, and consent obtained verbally. Verbal consent after full explanation is obtained for studies which are perhaps comparisons of various proven and frequently used treatments (Fig. 17/1). Any research which involves the use of specialised techniques, new drugs, or different from 'normal' methods of administering drugs, requires that the patient gives *written* consent for the trial, as well as verbal.

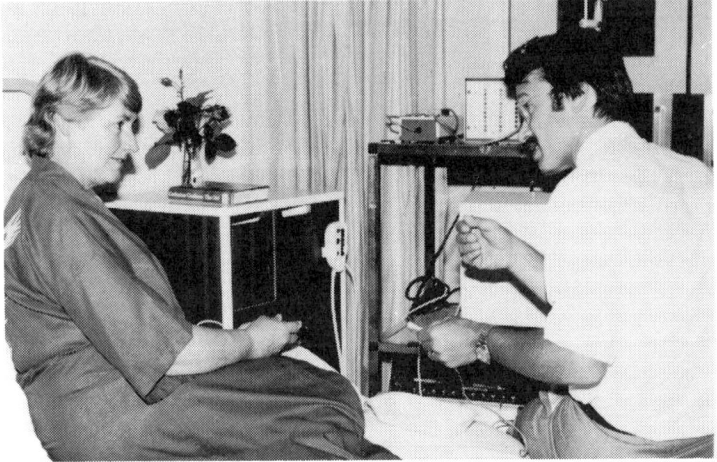

Fig. 17/1   Pre-operative explanation. The researcher must ensure that the patient is fully aware of the nature and purpose of the trial, and what is involved. This patient is being taught, pre-operatively, how to use the electronic linear visual analogue

THE NURSE'S ROLE – BEING THERE

In hospital, all proposed medical research has to be put before the hospital ethical committee. Research as an activity, just as nursing as an activity, has its own ethical code of practice which must be observed by the researcher. Patients have a right to expect a recognised code of conduct from the professional nurse, and nurses have a right to expect a recognised code of conduct from the researcher who wishes to undertake research in the area for which she is responsible. It is therefore important that the nurse, in giving access to a researcher, is aware of certain points, even if she is not directly involved. The nurse working on a surgical ward where acute pain research is undertaken, is entitled to be informed about the aim and purpose of the research, and whether there is any risk or inconvenience to the participating patients or ward staff. Moreover, she should assure herself that respect for confidentiality is maintained.

It is the responsibility of the researcher to explain the research to all the people involved in it, and to provide any requested information. When ward nurses are unaware of what is going on, they are placed in a position of doubt and difficulty. A chance remark made by an uninformed nurse may cause unnecessary anxiety to the patient by the communication of her own doubts about the proposed treatment.

BEING ACTIVELY INVOLVED

Nurses who are actively involved in pain research may be working with doctors, or on their own. The nurse who assists in research may have total responsibility for the execution of the research, or she may play a specific part, great or small, in it. Being involved in research is perhaps the most effective introduction to research activity. The collection of data by nurses for medical research has the potential of being most useful in gaining an insight into all aspects of research. The ward nurse who agrees to assist, must be very sure of her role in the research and should not agree to carry out a task for which she is not competent. Any nurse participating in a research project should be aware, not only of the aims and objectives of the study, but also the methods and means by which the required data are to be collected. This will involve scrutiny of the research protocol, which should be made available for all staff to read and for reference.

Communication is a vital role and responsibility of nurses who are actively involved with patients who are taking part in research. Communication about the study is necessary and important if it is to go smoothly. Everyone needs to know what is happening, what needs to be done, and not done, and also when the study is completed. Sometimes the research will involve other personnel or hospital departments who must be informed, so that necessary procedures will be carried out in a way that does not interfere with the study. This can all take a great deal of time, and could mean that the (medical) researcher requires an assistant, who may be a trained nurse.

When a clinical research nurse is available she may be responsible for the care of the patient before, and during, the study, ensuring that the ward staff are informed and aware of all aspects of the research. It would be the clinical research nurse's responsibility to liaise with other disciplines or departments and she might also be responsible for the selection of suitable candidates for the study.

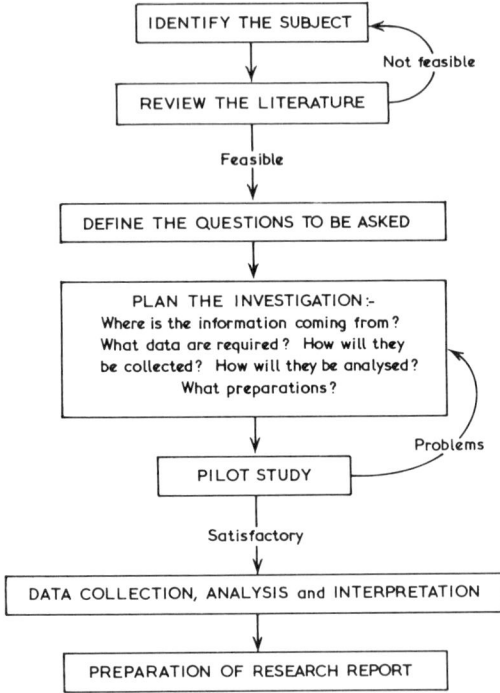

Fig. 17/2   The research process

DOING THE RESEARCH

Any nurse undertaking research of her own, needs to have an understanding of the research process (Fig. 17/2). The first step in the research process is to identify the subject and purpose of the study. The purpose of research is to acquire new knowledge, so, the question that must be asked before embarking on a study, is 'what can be learned from it'?

Having identified a suitable problem to be researched, the chosen subject needs to be explored to give insight into the reality and feasibility of undertaking such a study. A critical review of available literature must first be undertaken, together with an assessment of the time required by the study, and the expertise and money needed.

If the proposed research is possible and meaningful, then the next step is to plan the investigation by choosing the design of the research. The method of investigation must be appropriate to the chosen study. At this stage the way in which information is to be collected, and the way in which it will be analysed has to be considered. The tools for collection of the facts to be recorded, known as data, must also be appropriate. If a descriptive study is planned, with the data collected by questionnaire and analysed by computer, then the design of the questionnaire must be suitable for computer analysis. In this situation advice from a computer programmer would be invaluable; another study might require help from a statistician at the planning stage.

Once the design of the study and method of data collection have been decided, the researcher must then make preparations. This may involve obtaining permission from an ethical committee or senior nursing and medical staff. The researcher must also ensure that information about the study is given to those who will be concerned with it.

Most research is tested by a pilot study. This is a small replica of the proposed study and enables the research method to be tried out. The pilot study may bring to light alterations that need to be made before the main study is undertaken.

Once the preliminary steps have been successfully achieved, then the full-scale data collection can begin. This should be the most straightforward part of the research, but there are pitfalls and hiccups – frequently more time is taken than had been anticipated, often for reasons outside the researcher's control.

Having collected the information, it must then be analysed according to the chosen method. Finally, interpretation of the findings and the conclusions of the research must be presented in a written research report.

METHODS USED TO ASSESS THE EFFECTIVENESS OF POSTOPERATIVE PAIN CONTROL

Assessment of pain and the effectiveness of any treatment is not easy. Accurate assessment has to be objective, but pain is subjective.

Pain, particularly associated with upper abdominal and thoracic surgery, will have a significant effect on the patient's ability to breathe normally. From this arises one objective method of assessing the effects of pain through monitoring respiratory function.

Recording of vital capacity (VC) may be undertaken pre-operatively and at intervals in the postoperative period. Measurements recorded are the forced expiratory volume in one second (FEV_1) and the forced vital capacity (FVC) using a spirometer. A peak flow meter records the peak expiratory flow rate (PEFR) in litres/second. Comparisons are made between pre- and postoperative recordings. Good pain control will show better respiratory function postoperatively than when pain is inadequately relieved.

Subjective estimation of the pain being experienced by the patient can be achieved by the use of rating scales. These may take the form of descriptive words giving the patient a range to choose from (Fig. 17/3). The characteristics of the pain sensation may not exactly

```
   Tick the box which describes the pain you have experienced since
   the last recording

1.  No pain                          [   ]

2.  Slight pain                      [   ]

3.  Moderate pain                    [   ]

4.  Severe pain                      [   ]

5.  The worst pain imaginable        [   ]
```

Fig. 17/3   A descriptive word rating scale for severity of pain

fit the words offered, as interpretation of language differs with individuals which may make it difficult for the patient to select the appropriate word.

A linear visual analogue is also subjective but a more specific method of recording the amount of pain being experienced by the patient (see Fig. 4/1, p. 46).

When used in the immediate postoperative period, this system is difficult for the patient alone. If filled in with the help of a nurse or a researcher, responses may be unwittingly influenced. Therefore, this form of recording has been modified and expanded by the use of an electronic device which enables the patient constantly to display and record his own ratings of pain, nausea and sedation (Welchew, 1982).

A hand-set is placed beside the patient who by pushing the slides on the hand-set illuminates an appropriate number of lights on an adjacent box. A continuous recording of the lights is made automatically on graph paper.

Patients are asked to change the ratings whenever they are aware of any change themselves. A button on the hand-set is operated when the light appears on the box at regular intervals. This is recorded and, when reading the graphs, one is assured that the patient was awake and that the records are likely to be accurate. By this means, the amount of pain, nausea and sedation that a patient felt is shown by his use of the analogue.

The amount of analgesic required by an individual to relieve pain in the postoperative period can be monitored by the use of sophisticated apparatus. The on-demand analgesic computer (ODAC) records each dose requested by the patient, thus providing a record for demand analgesia over a given period of time. This record, both of the amount of drug consumed, and the times of demand, can be compared with the electronic linear visual analogue scales for pain, sedation and nausea. A picture of individual patient requirement for a particular drug together with the effects of that drug emerges. Individual patients may form a series and the findings from one group of patients may be compared with another who are given a different drug by the same system of administration.

METHODS USED TO EVALUATE PAIN-RELIEVING DRUGS

Evaluation of drugs under trial can be undertaken objectively by 'blinding' the trial. In a single blind study, the patient will be unaware of the type of analgesic received, although the researcher will know that Group A receives one drug, Group B another. Comparisons can be made between the responses to the drugs of two groups.

In a double-blind trial, neither the researcher nor the patient knows which of the two drugs are being given – in this case, all the preparations will be specially packed to look alike and will be coded. As a rule, the groups will be randomly selected so that the researcher cannot expect a pattern to emerge. In some trials, placebos are used and a patient's response to a dummy drug compared to the response to actual medication. The use of such placebos in the field of acute pain management could raise ethical questions.

When new methods or new drugs are being evaluated, it is vital that accurate information be obtained. Nurses working on wards where studies are in progress may be asked to make additional observations for a variety of different reasons. It is very important that such observations are obtained accurately.

Two examples of the types of research undertaken for the study of acute pain are now described.

1. A CLINICAL TRIAL

A clinical trial is often designed to test the hypothesis that one drug can offer significantly better analgesia than another to which it is compared. The protocol of such a study, undertaken by the authors, follows.

A double-blind comparison of sublingual buprenorphine versus intramuscular morphine in the treatment of moderate postoperative pain

Background
Buprenorphine is a relatively new analgesic which exhibits both partial agonist and antagonist properties. It is novel in having very slow drug-receptor kinetics which allow it to have a long duration of action while maintaining low blood levels. It has been suggested that sublingual buprenorphine offers the potential of potent analgesia of long duration and fewer side-effects than other routes of administration. In addition the sublingual route offers the advantage of being totally non-painful compared with the more conventional intramuscular route.

This trial has been designed to test the hypothesis that sublingual buprenorphine can offer significantly better analgesia with fewer side-effects than the standard postoperative narcotic morphine, when both are given in a randomised double-blind manner, 6-hourly for moderate postoperative pain.

Patient selection
Patients admitted to the trial will include:

1. Those presenting for elective non-cancer, non-urgent surgery
2. Patients aged between 20 and 65 years of age
3. Patients in the American Society of Anestheologists (ASA) gradings (for fitness for anaesthesia) I and II

4. Patients who have given their informed consent to participate
5. Patients whom the surgeon consents to admit to the trial.

Patients will be excluded from the trial if:

1. They are not in the above groups
2. They have a known sensitivity to the drugs used in the trial
3. They have a painful condition not related to the operative site
4. They are scheduled for thoracic, upper abdominal or other surgery known to cause severe postoperative pain
5. They have been given sedatives of any kind within 24 hours of the trial.

Ethics
The protocol for the trial will be submitted to the hospital ethical committee before instituting the trial.

Method of administration
Twenty patients admitted to the trial will be randomly allocated to one of two groups called A and B. Both groups of patients will be given a standard premedication and anaesthetic for their operation.

The trial will commence as soon as each patient wakes from anaesthesia and asks for analgesia. The trial will end 24 hours later. Group A patients will be given an intramuscular injection of morphine (10mg/70kg body-weight) and a sublingual placebo tablet every 6 hours for the first 24 hours after operation.

Group B patients will receive an intramuscular injection of 0.3mg of buprenorphine and a sublingual placebo at the start of the trial period, followed by an intramuscular saline placebo and 0.4mg sublingual buprenorphine every 6 hours.

The identities of the two groups will be kept in a sealed envelope on the ward and also in pharmacy. The identities will not be known by the doctors and nurses treating the patients unless the sealed envelopes are opened in an emergency or at the end of the trial.

Assessment
1. The patients will make continuous observations on an electronic linear visual analogue system for pain, sedation and nausea during the whole of the 24-hour trial.
2. Respiratory function tests, including the PEFR, the FEV_1, and the FVC, will be performed pre-operatively and at 18 and 24 hours postoperatively.

3. Observations of the patients' fluid intake and output will be recorded during the period of study.
4. At the end of the study each patient will be asked to make observations on linear visual analogues of pain for his average pain level and maximum pain level during the period of study.

Calculations
1. Graphs of the mean pain, sedation and nausea scores expressed by each group will be drawn against the corresponding time post-operatively.
2. The mean total pain, sedation and nausea scores for each group will be calculated and the significance of their difference calculated.
3. The mean postoperative respiratory function tests will be calculated at 18 and 24 hours postoperatively for each group and the significance of the differences between the groups calculated.
4. The mean postoperative fluid intake and output of the two groups will be calculated and the significance of their difference found.
5. The group means of the average and maximum pain scores will be calculated and the significance of their difference found.

Anaesthetic management
All patients in each group will be premedicated with 30ml Magnesium Trisilicate Mixture BP orally, immediately before coming to theatre. Anaesthesia will be induced with a sleep dose of Althesin, followed by 66% nitrous oxide in oxygen and an anaesthetic concentration of halothane, with the patients breathing spontaneously through a mask.

Preparing for the trial
Considerable preparations were required during the planning stage of this trial. So that all the drugs looked alike, specially prepared ampoules and tablets were obtained from the manufacturer. These were held by the hospital pharmacy who issued instructions to all nurses and doctors concerned with the trial (Table 1).

The reason for both the groups having tablets and injections was twofold. First, had the two groups received either/or, then the patients, nurses, and researcher would have known immediately, as the preparations, both in appearance, and administration, were quite different from each other. Second, while some patients might feel that tablets could not be as strong as injections, others might be biased in favour of tablets because of a dislike of injections.

Patients admitted to this trial were given a very full explanation of the protocol. Each was told that if, at any time during the 24 hours of the study, they should become dissatisfied with the pain-relief, then the study would be discontinued. In the event, one patient, after his second injection and tablets, asked to change to a different medication. He was immediately withdrawn from the trial and prescribed alternative medication by the duty house officer.

During the investigation, instructions were written in the nursing files and on the drug Kardex regarding treatment for nausea if it occurred. As it was the side-effects of the two drugs that were being monitored, it was important that these were influenced as little as possible by the addition of drugs which might interfere with such effects.

A copy of the protocol was attached to the patient's notes for the duration of the trial so that all the information was readily available to anyone who might need it.

Table 1 Nursing instructions for the sublingual buprenorphine vs. intramuscular morphine trial

When informed of a new patient entering into the trial:

1. Order a trial treatment pack from the Pharmacy on the next page of your Controlled Drug order book.
2. Enter the patient's full name and registration number on the Controlled Drug order.
3. During the trial period, all trial material must be treated as Controlled Drugs.
4. Administer the doses at the exact specified times and in the correct dose order (please read ampoule labels and tablet bottle labels carefully for this information):

Time	Dose Number	Drugs to be administered together
0 hours	1	10mg morphine IM + 2 × 0.2mg sublingual tablets buprenorphine
6 hours	2	10mg morphine IM + 2 × 0.2mg sublingual tablets buprenorphine
12 hours	3	repeat as before
18 hours	4	repeat as before
24 hours	End of trial – refer to drug Kardex for further treatment.	

5. For each patient, record exact administration times on the appropriate Controlled Drug record sheet (included in each treatment pack).
6. Keep this record sheet with the patient's drug Kardex during the trial period.
7. Hand in the completed record sheet to Miss X at the end of the trial.
8. For further information contact:

2. A SURVEY BY QUESTIONNAIRE (see p. 164)

A survey normally covers a large number of subjects in an enquiry. This may be undertaken by using a questionnaire on which the patient records the answers himself. These answers describe an existing situation and are therefore providing information which has not in any way been influenced by the researcher.

The authors undertook a descriptive study of postoperative pain, the objective being to correlate postoperative analgesic drugs and regimes with quality of analgesia in patients who were not in the artificial environment of controlled trials. Data were collected from 1053 patients.

A two-part questionnaire was devised. Permission was obtained from four consultant surgeons to approach their postoperative patients on four different wards. The first part of the questionnaire was answered by patients on the day they left hospital, following any operation. This provided the opinions which they were likely to take home with them after their various forms of therapy. The second part of the form was filled in by the research nurse. Using nursing and medical records, she recorded the details of their postoperative medication, type of surgery performed, and other relevant details.

A pilot study, when analysed, revealed gaps in the required information, additional questions were added before the main data collection took place. Patients were approached by the research nurse, who was not a member of the ward team, and asked if they would fill in a questionnaire about their operations. They were told that many of the questions related to pain that they might have suffered, and they were assured that the information was confidential and would not be seen by the doctors or nurses who had looked after them.

The whole questionnaire was designed for computer analysis and so required that the patients put a cross in the appropriate box for each answer. On completion of the questionnaire each was placed in a pre-addressed sealed envelope and returned to the researcher by internal hospital mail.

REFERENCE

Welchew, E. A. (1982). A postoperative pain recorder. *Anaesthesia*, **37**, 838–41.

QUESTIONNAIRE RELATING TO THE ABOVE SURVEY

Name ....

THANK YOU FOR YOUR HELP

The information on this questionnaire is strictly confidential.

It will be grouped together with similar information from many other patients, and no permanent record of the patients' names or identities will be kept.

No part of it will be seen by the doctors and nurses working on the wards.

POSTOPERATIVE PATIENT QUESTIONNAIRE

Card [1] 1

1. HOSP. NUMBER ▮☐☐☐☐ 2,3,4,5
2. AGE ☐☐ 6,7
3. DATE OF OP. ☐☐☐☐☐☐ 8,9,10,11,12,13

THE FOLLOWING QUESTIONS ARE TO BE ANSWERED BY
THE PATIENT

(please put a *cross* in the correct answer's box)

5. Have you ever had major surgery before? YES ☐ 14
   NO ☐ 15

6. Were you told enough *before* your operation about YES ☐ 16
   what would happen to you during your stay here? NO ☐ 17

7. Before your operation what did you
   expect the pain afterwards to be like? NO PAIN AT ALL ☐ 18
   MILD PAIN ☐ 19
   MODERATE PAIN ☐ 20
   SEVERE PAIN ☐ 21
   VERY SEVERE PAIN ☐ 22
   THE WORST PAIN IMAGINABLE ☐ 23

8. Were you told that strong pain-killers would be YES ☐ 24
   readily available after your operation? NO ☐ 25

9. Were you given postoperative pain-killers? YES ☐ 26
   NO ☐ 27

10. Did the pain-killers work?

YES ☐	28
NO ☐	29
NOT APPLICABLE ☐	30

11. Were you given pain-killers as often as you felt that you needed them?

YES ☐	31
NO ☐	32
NOT APPLICABLE ☐	33

12. Do you think that you were sometimes given pain-killers when you did not need them?

YES ☐	34
NO ☐	35
NOT APPLICABLE ☐	36

13. If you were not given pain-killers, do you think that they would have helped to make you more comfortable?

YES ☐	37
NO ☐	38
NOT APPLICABLE ☐	39

14. Did you have more or less postoperative pain than you expected?

MORE ☐	40
LESS ☐	41

15. What was the AVERAGE pain level for the first day after your operation?

NO PAIN AT ALL ☐	42
MILD PAIN ☐	43
MODERATE PAIN ☐	44
SEVERE PAIN ☐	45
VERY SEVERE PAIN ☐	46
THE WORST PAIN IMAGINABLE ☐	47

16. What was the average degree of pain relief obtained from your pain-killers?

NOT APPLICABLE ☐	48
NO RELIEF AT ALL ☐	49
VERY LITTLE PAIN RELIEF ☐	50
MODERATE PAIN RELIEF ☐	51
ALMOST COMPLETE PAIN RELIEF ☐	52
COMPLETE PAIN RELIEF ☐	53

17. Did you dislike being so SLEEPY after your operation?

YES ☐	54
NO ☐	55

18. Did you suffer from NAUSEA or VOMITING?

YES ☐	56
NO ☐	57

19. Did you suffer from ITCHING after your operation?   YES ☐   58   NO ☐   59

20. Were you DIZZY after your operation?   YES ☐   60   NO ☐   61

21. Did you feel WEAK after your operation?   YES ☐   62   NO ☐   63

22. Did you find INJECTIONS painful?   YES ☐   64   NO ☐   65

23. Did you find HAVING BLOOD TAKEN painful?   YES ☐   66   NO ☐   67

24. Did you find PHYSIOTHERAPY painful?   YES ☐   68   NO ☐   69

25. Did you find changing wound dressings or removal of stitches or drains painful?   YES ☐   70   NO ☐   71

26. Did you find BED BATHS painful?   YES ☐   72   NO ☐   73

FOR OFFICE USE ONLY

Card ☐ 1
HOSPITAL No.■■ ☐☐☐ 2,3,4,5

1st ANALGESIC
A. Name code   ☐☐ 6,7
B. Dose code   ☐☐ 8,9
C. No. of doses given   ☐☐ 10,11
D. Analgesic technique code   ☐☐ 12,13
E. Time after surgery of last dose (hrs)   ☐☐☐ 14,15,16

2nd ANALGESIC
F. Name code   ☐☐ 17,18
G. Dose card   ☐☐ 19,20
H. No. of doses given   ☐☐ 21,22
I. Analgesic technique code   ☐☐ 22,24
J. Time after surgery of last dose (hrs)   ☐☐☐ 25,26,27

K. Open ended DDA prescription?
    (N=0, Y=1) ☐ 28
L. Written in correct part of form
    (N=0, Y=1) ☐ 29
M. Was prescription obeyed?
    (N=0, Y=1) ☐ 30
N. If NOT, was it given more (1) or less (0) ☐ 31
    frequently?
O. Anti-emetic name code. ☐ 32
P. How many doses given? ☐☐ 33,34

RESPIRATORY FUNCTION TESTS

    Preop   FEV^1 ☐☐ 35,36
              FVC ☐☐ 37,38
              PEFR ☐☐☐ 39,40,41
    Postop. 1 FEV^1 ☐☐ 42,43
              FVC ☐☐ 44,45
              PEFR ☐☐☐ 46,47,48
    Postop. 2 FEV^1 ☐☐ 49,50
              FVC ☐☐ 51,52
              PEFR ☐☐☐ 53,54,55

Q. Operation code ☐☐ 56,57
R. Gender (F=0, M=1) ☐☐ 58,59
S. Entonox given? (N=0, Y=1) ☐☐ 60,61
T. Ward (H1 = 1, H2 = 2, K1/2 = 0) ☐☐ 62,63
                                     ☐☐ 64,65

                                     ☐☐ 66,67
                                     ☐☐ 68,69
                                     ☐☐ 70,71

FURTHER READING

Bond, M. R. (1979). *Pain: Its Nature, Analysis and Treatment.* Churchill Livingstone, Edinburgh.

Budd, K. (1984) *Pain.* Update Publications, London.

Davitz, J. R. and Davitz, L. L. (1981). *Inferences of Patients' Pain and Psychological Distress: Studies of Nursing Behaviours.* Springer Publishing Company, New York.

Fairley, P. (1978). *The Conquest of Pain.* Michael Joseph, London.

Jacox, A. (1977). *Measurement of Clinical Pain: A Source Book for Nurses and Other Health Professionals.* Little Brown and Co, Boston.

McCaffery, M. (1983). *Nursing the Patient in Pain.* Harper and Row, London.

MacLeod Clark, J. and Hockey, L. (1979). *Research for Nursing: A Guide for the Enquiring Nurse.* HM+M Publishers Ltd, Aylesbury.

Melzack, R. (1973). *The Puzzle of Pain.* Penguin Education, Harmondsworth.

Sofaer, B. (1984). *Pain: a Handbook for Nurses.* Harper and Row, London.

INDEX